AIDS

CRISIS CONTROL IN UGANDA

AIDS
CRISIS CONTROL IN UGANDA

The Use of HAART

Dorothy J. N. Kalanzi

CAMBRIA PRESS

Amherst, New York

Requests for permission should be directed to:
permissions@cambriapress.com, or mailed to:
Cambria Press
20 Northpointe Parkway, Suite 188
Amherst, NY 14228

Library of Congress Cataloging-in-Publication Data

Kalanzi, Dorothy J.
AIDS crisis control in Uganda: the use of HAART / Dorothy J. Kalanzi.
p.; cm.
Includes bibliographical references and index.
ISBN 978-1-60497-787-5
I. Title.
[DNLM: 1. Acquired Immunodeficiency Syndrome—drug therapy—Uganda.
2. HIV Infections—drug therapy—Uganda.
3. Anti-HIV Agents—therapeutic use—Uganda.
4. Antiretroviral Therapy, Highly Active—Uganda. WC 503.2]

362.19697920096761—dc23

2011040693

This book is dedicated to
my late beloved father, Andrew Kalibbala Kalanzi;
my mother, Justine Wangabira Kalanzi;
my late sister, Millica Kyazze Kalanzi,
whose untimely death inspired me to do research on HIV/AIDS;
my brother, Joel Sewanyana; and Africa.

Table of Contents

List of Tables

ACKNOWLEDGMENTS

All glory is to God, who orders my steps in the successful endeavors of my dreams. Without His grace, I would accomplish nothing. Secondly, I would like to thank my late beloved father, Andrew Kalibbala Kalanzi, and mother, Justine Wangabira Kalanzi. Thank you for helping me access a good education in Africa, both at home and in school, that empowered me with skills to write this book.

To my late sister and best friend, Millica Kyazze Kalanzi, who died of AIDS in 1997. The love we cherished over the years and her untimely death inspired me to do research on AIDS. May her soul rest in peace.

I would also like to thank Dr. James Williams, Dr. Ami Moore, Dr. Joseph Oppong, and Dr. Abigail Tilton for their guidance in the initial phases of writing this book.

I also thank Captain Dr. Godfrey Bwiire, Dr. Joseph Mwebe, Julliana K. Nyombi, Sikora Okure, Dr. Cissy Kityo, and my brother, Joel Sewanyana Kalanzi, for their assistance during the data collection process. To my friends Ester Taylor, Inshirah Nabhan, Rubye M. Dodson, and Lynne R. Barga, and my sister Susan Kalanzi, thank you for your support.

Most importantly, to the people enrolled in the highly active antiretroviral therapy (HAART) who shared experiences with HIV treatment amid physical, psychological, and emotional distress, thank you. This book would not have been completed without your participation. Your input may contribute to improvements in the treatment of AIDS.

AIDS
CRISIS CONTROL IN UGANDA

Chapter 1

Introduction

Three decades since the initial diagnosis, AIDS remains one of the most complex health challenges, a signature disease of the present age (Robbins, 2005). It began as an epidemic. However, by 2000, AIDS had reached all corners of the world and had been declared a pandemic by the World Health Organization (WHO) (Joint United Nations Program on HIV/AIDS [UNAIDS], 2006b). It is estimated that 33.3 million individuals around the world are currently living with the virus, the majority of whom scholars predict will prematurely die from AIDS-related conditions (Bongaarts, Pelletier, & Gerland, 2009). Since the beginning of the epidemic, it is estimated that more than 60 million people around the world have been infected with the virus and nearly 30 million have died from the disease (WHO, 2011a). This puts AIDS at the top of the list of the most destructive pandemics in the history of mankind. Despite efforts to curb the spread of the disease, the infection rate around the world continues to rise. In 2009 there were 2.6 million newly infected cases worldwide. AIDS does not discriminate against geographical space, social class, gender, or age. However, as is the pattern for all illnesses, vulnerable population groups, such as those at the bottom of the social stratification system—the poor, women, and children—have been disproportionately affected by HIV/AIDS. Statistics reveal that since the epidemic outbreak, the poor (especially those living in low-income nations, specifically in sub-Saharan Africa) have carried the biggest burden of AIDS. This may be because, unlike in developed nations where the infection rate was easily contained in the first few years after the initial outbreak, the disease spread like fire in developing countries that lacked well-established surveillance, monitoring, and prevention systems. Of the 33 million individuals living with the virus in 2009, about 23 million lived in sub-Saharan Africa (71%) (UNAIDS, 2009). Only about 1.5 million lived in the United States and Canada combined. During the same year, sub-Saharan Africa reported about 1.8 million new HIV infections as opposed to the 70,000 reported in North America (UNAIDS, 2009). Likewise, of the 1.8 million individuals who died of HIV/AIDS worldwide in 2009, 1.3 million are said to have been living in sub-Saharan Africa as opposed to the 26,000 in North America (WHO, 2011b). The advent of antibiotics in the 1940s had steadily increased life expectancy globally by 1980 to above 60. However, AIDS has tremendously reduced life expectancy, specifically in countries most affected by the pandemic as compared to the least affected. For example, the average life expectancy of individuals who live in sub-Saharan Africa is about 54 years. In contrast, life expectancy in developed countries remains high—with that of Japan being 86, Australia, 84, and the United States, 79 (UNAIDS, 2010a).

Females, especially those of childbearing age (15–45), have also been disproportionately infected with the disease. According to the World Health Organization and the Joint United Nations Program on HIV/AIDS estimates, in 2009 some 50% of those living with HIV/AIDS globally were females (Laing & Hodgkin, 2006; UNAIDS, 2006c). In sub-Saharan Africa, females carried 60% of the HIV/AIDS burden in 2009 (WHO, 2011b). In a study of nine countries in sub-Saharan Africa, Gouws (2008) reported an HIV prevalence rate of about three times higher for females as opposed to males ages 15–24. The most affected population groups, especially in terms of age and gender, raise public health concerns, one of which is the potential of passing the virus from mother to child during childbirth (Esu-Williams & Blancard, 2002; Weinberg & Friedland, 1998). Global surveillance statistics show that 1,200 children under age 15 were being infected daily with the virus in 2008 alone, of which 90% lived in resource-constrained nations such as those of sub-Saharan Africa (WHO, 2009a).

Despite the aggravated attack of AIDS on the world population as just illustrated, there have been remarkable innovations in the successful control and treatment of AIDS. As detailed later, the introduction and to a greater extent the successful implementation of highly active antiretroviral therapy (HAART) have exonerated those infected with the virus from an AIDS-related automatic death sentence to healthier and extended longevity—if they adhere to medication regimens as well as to healthy lifestyles that reduce the risk of HIV infection, such as abstinence from sex, having only one sex partner, or the regular use of condoms. On the contrary, HAART adherence failure and unsafe sexual practices may undermine public health efforts to control HIV/AIDS morbidity and mortality. This may be particularly true in low-income nations such as those in sub-Saharan Africa, many of which have seen increasing access to HAART since the beginning of the millennium. As elaborated later, this study explores HAART adherence and the effect of anti-HIV drugs on individuals suffering from HIV/AIDS in Uganda.

Defining HIV and AIDS

HIV stands for human immunodeficiency virus. It is a retrovirus that enters humans and destroys the immune system, causing AIDS. AIDS stands for acquired immunodeficiency syndrome, and it is the final stage of HIV infection. It is not inherited but acquired after birth with the destruction of the immune system. AIDS is not a single disease but a syndrome diagnosed after manifestations of a number of illnesses that typically affect individuals with weakened immune systems or individuals with a CD4 cell count of 200 or less. CD4 cells are a type of immune system cells that help the body to fight disease. A normal person is expected to have a CD4 cell count of about between 600 and 1,200. Anyone with AIDS has HIV. However, one may have HIV without having AIDS. HIV/AIDS may be better understood with a description of disease progression that results from the destruction of CD4 cells. That is, after HIV enters the human body, it needs to make copies of itself. Because HIV is a retrovirus, it can only replicate itself within a host's cell. Therefore, in order to make copies of itself, HIV chooses and enters the CD4 cell (sometimes referred to as the T-cell), destroying it in the process of replication. When HIV enters the body and begins to destroy the CD4 cells, disease progression partially characterized by the CD4 cell count is often grouped in four stages based on clinical standards. The first stage begins at HIV infection, and it may last for a few weeks. This stage is usually characterized by manifestations of flu-like symptoms. During this stage, the HIV viral load is high, but the immune system is strong and it normally responds to the CD4 cell destruction by producing antibodies to fight the virus. As the virus continues to destroy the CD4 cells, HIV infection progresses to the clinical asymptomatic stage, which may last as long as 10 years based on one's health, sexual lifestyle, and economic status. For instance, disease progression from HIV to AIDS may be faster if the infected has other poor health conditions, engages in unsafe sexual practices such as having sex with multiple partners without regularly using a condom, or lacks access to a good diet. During the second stage, no significant symptoms are manifested, and although the destruction of the CD4 cells continues, antibodies continue to fight off HIV. Continuous destruction of the CD4 cells by HIV leads to stage 3, referred to as the symptomatic stage, in which the CD4 cell count may have fallen to about between 350 and 200. During this stage, the immune system can no longer keep up with the fight against the HIV destruction of the CD4 cells or other illnesses as a result of years of deterioration. This is when symptoms, some of which may be severe, begin to be manifested as opportunistic illnesses. Some of the symptoms during stage 3 include but are not limited to severe weight loss, chronic diarrhea, persistent fever, persistent oral candidiasis, oral hairy leukoplakia, pulmonary tuberculosis, herpes zoster, and fungal nail infections. These conditions may also be manifested in the final stage of the disease. Stage 4 is the final stage of HIV progression, at which point an individual is diagnosed with AIDS. The immune system at this stage is so weak—with a CD4 cell count of 200 or less—that it can no longer fight infectious illnesses. Stage 4 is manifested with severe opportunistic infections and cancers, such as pneumocystis carinii pneumonia (PCP), Kaposi's sarcoma, lymphoma, extrapulmonary tuberculosis, HIV wasting syndrome, esophageal candidiasis, invasive cervical carcinoma, central nervous system toxoplasmosis, and chronic isosporiasis, to name only a few. Several of these illnesses might be manifested at once or individually. Without treatment, HIV/AIDS leads to death. As illustrated further on, it was the manifestation of some of these listed opportunistic illnesses that led to the initial discovery of AIDS.

Discovery of HIV

AIDS was first diagnosed in the United States in 1981 among five homosexual men in San Francisco and New York who portrayed manifestations of PCP and Kaposi's sarcoma (Bongaarts, 1996; Fannin, Gottlieb, & Weisman, 1982; WebMD, 2008). PCP is caused by a fungus. Symptoms of PCP include a dry cough, fever, difficulty breathing, shortness of breath, weight loss, and night sweats. Kaposi's sarcoma is a type of cancer resulting in patches of tissue grown under the skin that look like mosquito bites. Overtime, tumors often develop in the mouth, nose, and gastrointestinal tract, affecting internal organs such as the stomach, liver, and lungs (Harden, 1992). PCP, Kaposi's sarcoma, and many other opportunistic illnesses are rare among healthy individuals but common among individuals with weakened immune systems, especially the elderly, premature children, malnourished individuals, and bone marrow or organ transplant recipients (Aliouat-Denis, 2008). Therefore, the discovery of these two conditions among population groups generally expected to be healthy was a mystery, and it raised public health concerns. Uncertainty about the new illness that led to manifestation of these health conditions triggered a wave of panic around the world with questions pertaining to its name, cause, mode of transmission, and treatment options. For example, because AIDS was first diagnosed among the gay community in the United States, in the early days it was generally thought to affect only homosexuals and thus named the gay-related immunodeficiency (GRID) (Gottlieb, 1981). Far from the United States and in the middle of sub-Saharan Africa, where the same disease was quietly but rapidly spreading, as the public watched large numbers of people become very ill and extremely skinny with manifestations of a multitude of opportunistic illnesses, one of which is referred to as the wasting syndrome before they died. The new disease was initially named *Slim* or *Mukenenya* by the Baganda in Uganda. *Mukenenya* means something that makes a person extremely thin or emaciated. Not until 1982 was "Acquired Immune Deficiency Syndrome" (AIDS) coined as the name for this new and mysterious illness (Harden, 1992). Currently, although individuals in Uganda know that it is AIDS, they still refer to it as *Slim* and *Mukenenya*.

Moreover, the naming of AIDS was followed by an urgent need to identify the disease-causing agent, which was necessary for prevention and treatment purposes. Among the many scientists around the world who focused on this endeavor were Dr. Luc Montagnier at the Pasteur Institute in France and Dr. Jay A. Levy at the University of California, San Francisco. They succeeded in the discovery of the type of retrovirus that causes AIDS in 1983, which Montagnier named the lymphadenopathy associated virus (LAV) and Levy the AIDS-associated retrovirus (ARV). Likewise, in 1984 Dr. Robert Gallo and scientists at the National Cancer Institute in the United States also discovered the two retroviruses that cause AIDS and named them HTLV-I and HTLV-II (Gottlieb, 1981). Controversy about the initial discovery of this agent arose. Mediated by the respective political heads of states for the United States and France at the time, the founding scientists agreed to share credit for what was considered the same discovery, and the AIDS-causing agent was given a common name in 1987, the human immunodeficiency virus (HIV) (Gottlieb, 1981).

Unfortunately, these discoveries did not ease public fears of AIDS because information about the mode of HIV exposure was still a mystery.

Because it was first diagnosed among homosexual men, AIDS was initially speculated to be caused by sin, specifically linked to homosexuality and promiscuity. Not until 1984 was it discovered that everyone was at risk of HIV infection because it was transmitted through exchange of fluids via various modes of exposure that include but are not limited to heterosexual intercourse, male-to-male sex, blood transfusion, mother-to-child transmission during childbirth, and intravenous drug use. The discovery that no one was immune to HIV infection generated panic within the public, which in turn led to prioritizing research for HIV control in developed nations such as the United States. By this time, further research on HIV had also led to the discovery of the HIV life cycle: soon after the virus enters the body, it targets the CD4 cell as its host, from where it begins to rapidly replicate itself, destroying the CD4 cell in the process. Equipped with this information, scientists quickly directed efforts toward the development of HIV treatment drugs (Brunton et al., 2006).

History of HIV Treatment

Anti-HIV drugs were first invented in the late 1980s (Deeks et al., 2003; Hammer et al., 2006; HIV Clinical Resource, 2007; Laing & Hodgkin, 2006; Palella et al., 1998). During the early stages of AIDS, the National Cancer Institute (NCI) led the search for HIV treatment. This may be attributed to the fact that the AIDS-causing agent (HIV) is a retroviral virus. Retroviruses attack the immune system cells directly rather than the body. Retroviruses cause not only illnesses such as AIDS but also cancers. In the fight against cancer, after the National Cancer Act was passed in 1971, the NCI had screened numerous antiretroviral compounds to treat cancer, many of which had completed clinical trials (Gottlieb, 1981). Therefore, when HIV was first discovered, the NCI already had potential retrovirus treatment compounds in stock, from which a choice was made to experiment treating HIV. Of the compounds in stock was zidovudine (AZT). Although it initially proved ineffective, AZT had been synthesized in 1964 by Jerome Horwitz and his colleagues at the Michigan Cancer Foundation to treat cancer (Saunders, 2000). A decade later, the same drug was tested and discovered to block the replication of retroviruses in mouse cells during Wolfram Ostertag's study at the Max Planck Institute in a search for an anti-Friend leukemia virus (FLV) drug (Gottlieb et al., 1981). The initial success of AZT against this specific retrovirus put it at the top of the list as a potential medicine to treat HIV in the 1980s. Dr. Samuel Broder, scientists at the NCI, and the GlaxoSmithKline company soon discovered that, although this drug did not kill HIV, it successfully suppressed its replication. Hence, AZT was to become the first drug approved and utilized in the treatment of HIV (Broder, 2010).

Noteworthy is the fact that, although experimentation with AZT began around 1983, the drug was not approved by the U.S. Food and Drug Administration (FDA) until 1987, after which it was named Retrovir (Broder, 2010). Using AZT to treat HIV did not come without challenges because it was a high risk for the development of drug-resistant HIV and the drug was highly toxic (Broder, 2010). Nevertheless, AZT's success in suppressing HIV replication enticed hope that AIDS could be controlled with medicine. AZT's approval by the FDA was an incentive for pharmaceutical companies around the world to develop newer and safer anti-HIV drugs. For instance, to focus on U.S. pharmaceutical companies, Hoffmann-La Roche manufactured Hivid, which was approved by the FDA in 1992 although soon discontinued. Bristol-Myers Squibb manufactured Zerit/stavudine, approved by the FDA in 1994. Hoffmann-La Roche manufactured Invirase, FDA approved in 1995. Abbott Laboratories' Norvir/ritonavir was approved by the FDA in 1996 (Flexner, 2007). Boehringer Ingelheim discovered nevirapine, which was approved by the FDA in 1996 (de Béthune, 2009). GlaxoSmithKline manufactured Combivir, a combination drug of lamivudine and zidovudine that the FDA approved in 1997. The Janssens Foundation and Tibotec researchers discovered etravirine, FDA approved in 2008 (de Béthune, 2009). Other U.S.-based drug manufacturing companies include Agouron Pharmaceuticals, Merck & Co., Inc., and Pfizer. As in the United States, there are various pharmaceutical companies around the world—including two Indian companies, namely Cipla and Ranbaxy—that manufacture generic anti-HIV drugs. As the public remains optimistic about a cure for HIV/AIDS, pharmaceutical companies continue to venture new medication innovations that may completely destroy the virus.

Anti-HIV Treatment Drugs

Currently, more than 25 different types of HIV antiretroviral drugs have been innovated and approved by the U.S. FDA (AIDS*info*, 2008; Hanson & Hicks, 2006; Laing & Hodgkin, 2006; Palella et al., 1998; Yeni et al., 2005). These drugs are grouped into six classes, namely nucleoside reverse transcriptase inhibitors (NRTIs), non-nucleoside reverse transcriptase inhibitors (NNRTIs), protease inhibitors (PIs), fusion inhibitors, integrase inhibitors, and entry inhibitors (AIDS InfoNet, 2011; Department of Health and Human Services [DHHS], 2007; McNicholl, 2007). Anti-HIV drugs' regimen dosages usually constitute three drugs from at least two different classes, and they target specific stages of the HIV lifecycle, which begins and is completed within the CD4 cell. Each drug blocks continuation of the replication process at a designated stage in the HIV lifecycle (de Béthune, 2009). For example, drugs that belong to the entry inhibitor class are utilized to prevent HIV from entering or attaching itself to the CD4 cell, which is the first stage of replication. The second stage is targeted by the NRTIs and NNRTIs, which prevent HIV from making its new DNA from its RNA by blocking the enzyme known as reverse transcriptase (de Béthune, 2009). Integrase inhibitors prevent HIV from integrating its newly formed DNA into the CD4 cell during the third stage. The fourth stage is targeted by PIs that hinder the protease enzyme from enabling completion of the HIV reproduction process. The three combination drugs commonly used to treat HIV include one NRTI, one NNRTI, and one PI (Tarby, 2004). Each dose combination is sometimes referred to as a cocktail (GlaxoSmithKline, 2008; Hammer et al., 2006). These combination drugs have somewhat reversed what may have been initially perceived by many global cultures as the curse of AIDS.

Downside of Anti-HIV Medication

Unfortunately, despite successful innovations and developments of existing antiretroviral drugs, challenges in the discovery of more effective and more efficient anti-HIV compounds that minimize public health concerns remain. First, anti-HIV drugs do not cure the disease but only slow the HIV replication process. Second, these drugs do not stop new HIV infection (Hanson & Hicks, 2006). Third, anti-HIV drugs are costly and inaccessible to those who may need them the most. Fourth, some of these drugs must be taken on an empty stomach and others on a full stomach, which is a contributor to poor adherence, especially for those who do not have access to a sufficient food supply (Cichocki, 2009). Fifth, once HAART treatment begins, drugs must be taken at the exact timing and in the right dosage, sometimes more than once a day as prescribed by the health care provider, which again contributes to adherence failure detailed later (Broder, 2010; Hanson & Hicks, 2006). Sixth, anti-HIV drugs may be toxic and cause numerous side effects. Side effects from anti-HIV drugs, some of which may be life threatening, include headache, dizziness, fatigue, problems with breathing, tingling, numbness, pain in the feet or hands, jaundice, aches, sensitivity to touch, liver or pancreas problems, diabetes, body fat deposits, fever, skin rash, blood in the urine, swelling of the feet, diarrhea, nausea, vomiting, stomach pain, and loss of appetite.

To minimize the public health challenges pertaining to anti-HIV medications, scientists and drug companies continue to devise ways to improve existing drugs or to develop newer and safer drugs (Sen et al., 2008). For example, unlike the earlier phases of HIV treatment that utilized one type of drug (such as AZT), to minimize the danger of the development of drug-resistant HIV, later treatment utilizes a combination of several different drugs taken in a single dose. Unfortunately, using different types of drugs to treat HIV means taking a number of pills per dose, often more than once a day. Research reveals pill burden as an influential factor for adherence failure, a major contributor to drug resistance. To improve adherence, some drug companies developed ways to combine two or more types of antiretroviral drugs in a single pill. This means that those in therapy can now take only one pill per dose and in some cases once a day instead of taking three or more pills in a single dose, as was the case in the earlier days of HIV treatment. For example, Atripla—manufactured by Bristol-Myers Squibb and Gilead Sciences—is one example of a multiclass combination caplet approved by the FDA in 2006; it combines three different drugs, namely efavirenz, emtricitabine, and tenofovir disoproxil fumarate (U.S. Department of State [USDS], 2011). Kaletra, approved by the FDA in 2000 and manufactured by Abbott Laboratories, is a combination of two different drugs—lopinavir and norvir—in one capsule. Combivir is a combination of lamivudine and zidovudine. Trizivir is a combination of abacavir, lamivudine, and zidovudine (Cichocki, 2009).

Another way that pharmaceutical companies have tried to minimize the problem of nonadherence and side effects is through the invention of enteric-coated drugs, such as Videx, developed by Bristol-Myers Squibb and approved by the FDA in 2000. Videx is not new, though; it was the second anti-HIV drug approved by the FDA in 1991. Discontinued since the invention of the new Videx enteric-coated pill, this compound was initially manufactured in a chewable tablet that dissolves in the stomach. One advantage of enteric-coated drugs is that they release the medication not in the stomach but after the capsule has reached the small intestines, which may decrease the risk of certain side effects, such as nausea (Cichocki, 2009). Another advantage to the new enteric-coated Videx is that it can also be taken only once a day, minimizing the pill burden problem (Cichocki, 2009). Although some of the newly innovated medications such as enteric-coated pills are not yet available to those receiving free HAART in low-income countries (as in Uganda), such efforts by pharmaceutical companies are making anti-HIV medications easier and safer to take than before, all of which may improve medication regimen adherence, which in turn may reduce the risk of the development of drug-resistant HIV. Minimizing this risk in low-income nations such as Uganda is crucial given the large numbers of those infected with the disease. Drug-resistant HIV is transmissible. If large numbers of people in low-income nations are infected with this strain, it may not easily be controlled by existing HIV drugs, which is a danger to public health.

HAART in Uganda

Because this study explores HAART adherence behavior in Uganda, it is important to give a brief background about the study area. Uganda is located in sub-Saharan East Africa, and it is about the size of the state of Oregon. The country occupies an area of approximately 93,070 square miles with a 2007 estimated population of 32 million people (USDS, 2008). The majority of people in Uganda live under the international poverty line, as evidenced by the 2009 national gross national income (GNI) per capita of $460 (U.S.) (World Bank, 2011). One of the reasons why Uganda was selected for this study is that it was one of the first nations to experience a very high HIV incidence, especially in the 1980s and 1990s. Although statistics do not exist, Uganda also had a drastic drop in the incidence of HIV/AIDS between the mid-1990s and the early 2000s (AVERTing, 2008). By 2006, it was estimated that 2 million Ugandans had been infected with HIV and about 1 million had died of AIDS-related causes (Uganda Ministry of Health, 2006). It remains a controversy as to when the first HIV case occurred in Uganda. However, it is speculated that despite the fact that HIV in Uganda was first diagnosed in two cases in 1982, the first incidences of HIV may have emerged soon after the 1978–1979 civil war that deposed Idi Amin Dada's political regime (Buve, Bishikwabo-Ssarhaza, & Mutangadura, 2002; AVERTing, 2008).

Although early HIV treatment in Uganda is not well documented, HAART was introduced in the United States and Uganda at about the same time (1996 and 1997, respectively). Unfortunately, the anti-HIV drug cost was so high that the majority of those affected in Uganda could not afford these drugs (MOH, 2003; Mugyenyi et al., 2006). By 2000, very few HAART-providing centers existed, and to the greatest extent they served a clique of Uganda's elite who could afford the cost of the drugs (MOH, 2003; UNAIDS, 2006c). Not until about 2004 were tens of thousands of marginalized Ugandans able to gain free access to these drugs through public programs funded by international organizations such as the WHO, World Bank, Global Fund, and the U.S.-based President's Emergency Plan for AIDS (PEPFAR) (Mugyenyi et al., 2006). Around the time this study was conducted, there were about 175 centers that provided free HAART to about 75,000 of the hundreds of thousands of individuals nationwide who had a diagnosis of full-blown AIDS and were on the brink of death (AVERTing, 2008; Hardon et al., 2006; WHO, 2006c). Of the 175 centers providing HAART in 2007, three centers located around Uganda's capital city were selected for this study. Two of those that participated in the study served about 3,200 civilians; the third center served about 1,000 soldiers and civilians. Although a few clients choose to travel from remote areas to access services at any of the centers under study, each of these centers serves individuals in the immediate surroundings of about a 75-kilometer radius.

HAART-providing centers in Uganda generally mimic those in the United States. However, several differences pertaining to the provision of services exist, basically as dictated by financial expense. To illustrate these differences, I will compare the three HAART-providing centers in Uganda under study with three centers in the United States: namely, the AIDS Services of North Texas (ASNT) in Denton, Texas; 360: Positive Care Center (PCC) in San Francisco, California; and the HIV Center at Northwestern Memorial Hospital in Chicago, Illinois.

The first difference is that free HAART in Uganda only became accessible to those who could not afford it at a cost in 2004. In contrast, the United States has been providing HAART to everyone who meets the access criterion (described later) since around 1996 (Hammer et al., 2006; The AIDS Support Organization [TASO], 2006). Additionally, HAART-providing centers in Uganda and the United States differ in terms of the recommended time to initiate taking anti-HIV drugs. Before discussing these differences, it is important to understand that the exact time at which to start anti-HIV drug treatment is not clear. It is also necessary to mention that study results associating HAART initiation time and the quality of life as based on staging of the disease are inconsistent (Gao, Nau, Rosenbluth, Scott, & Woodward, 2000). Some scholars have demonstrated that disease progression is greater in persons who start HAART with a CD4 cell count below 200 than in those starting therapy above this level (Garcia et al., 2004). However, Wood et al. (2003) compared benefits of HAART for individuals whose CD4 cell count was between 200 and 350 with those of persons whose CD4 cell count was below 200 and found that both groups equally benefited from treatment. Nevertheless, regardless of available information about when to initiate anti-HIV drugs, HAART initiation in Uganda (unlike in the United States) strictly follows the WHO guidelines and is based on clinical and immunological assessments, such as CD4 cell count and the manifestation of specific HIV/AIDS opportunistic illnesses as discussed later (WHO, 2003a; WHO, 2008c). For example, according to WHO (2004), free access to HAART in resource-constrained nations may only be initiated under one of three conditions. The first condition is a CD4 cell count of 200 or below, regardless of HIV disease progression stage (Daniels, 2005; WHO, 2008c). The second condition is that an individual has reached stage 3 of HIV, possesses a CD4 cell count of 350 or below, and has experienced any of the AIDS definitive illnesses, such as Kaposi's sarcoma, wasting syndrome, pulmonary tuberculosis, pneumonitis, lymphoma of the brain, recurrent invasive bacterial infections, persistent mucosal candidiasis, chronic diarrhea, or prolonged fever of unknown etiology (Daniels, 2005; Laing & Hodgkin, 2006; WHO, 2004). The third condition is that the individual has reached stage 4 of the disease or has been diagnosed with AIDS, irrespective of CD4 cell count or manifestation of any serious opportunistic illness (WHO, 2008c).

U.S. centers, on the contrary, follow the Department of Health and Human Services guidelines for initiation of anti-HIV drug treatment. These guidelines recommend that all HIV-positive expecting mothers and anyone with symptomatic HIV illnesses in the United States should initiate HAART regardless of CD4 cell count (Hammer et al., 2006; Sterling, Chaisson, Keruly, & Moore, 2003; Yeni et al., 2005). However, DHHS only recommends HAART initiation for asymptomatic individuals when one's CD4 cell count is 350 or below, a count higher than that of individuals in developing nations (Panel on Antiretroviral Guidelines for Adult and Adolescents [PAGAA], 2008; Sterling et al., 2003; Wood et al., 2003). Asymptomatic HIV-positive individuals in the United States with a CD4 cell count above 350 are discouraged, but not prevented, from starting HAART (Hammer et al., 2006).

Several reasons explain HAART initiation restriction guidelines both in Uganda and the United States. In reference to resource-constrained nations that strictly follow WHO's HAART access guidelines, restrictions may pertain to forces of demand and supply for highly active antiretroviral drugs. For instance, WHO's goal at the time this study was conducted was to treat everyone affected by 2010 (WHO, 2004). Millions of those affected who need free drugs live in developing nations. An economic implication in the provision of free HAART is that these drugs do not cure HIV but only suppress its replication, such that they must be administered for life once treatment is initiated (Hammer et al., 2006). WHO's dilemma is that the demand is high, yet a lifetime supply of these drugs for everyone in need is not possible because of the high cost. Therefore, in order to reach WHO's goal of free access of anti-HIV drugs to all in a given time frame, it is necessary to restrict availability of these drugs in resource-constrained nations by providing treatment only to those who need it the most.

Several reasons that explain the United States' DHHS-recommended HAART initiation guidelines also exist. For example, prior to 1998, the DHHS recommended treating anyone in the United States infected with HIV regardless of clinical status or disease progression stage. This policy was referred to as the "hit early and hit hard" strategy, and it was established because it was initially assumed HAART would cure HIV (AIDS*info*, 2008). However, after it was apparent that HIV had no cure and treatment was a life sentence, the "hit early and hit hard" HAART initiation policy was revised (Hammer et al., 2006). This was because the discovery that AIDS remained without a cure was followed by public health concerns pertaining to anti-HIV drug side effects and suboptimal adherence issues. Of major concern was the fact that starting HAART leads to significant adjustments in lifestyle that are often recommended to individuals under treatment, such as complying with a complex treatment regimen, changes in diet, and so forth, all of which may be challenging to the client whose treatment is for life. Failure to adhere to HAART lifestyle regimens may foster medication adherence failure (AIDS*info*, 2008). Suboptimal HAART adherence is a public health concern because of the potential for the development of a drug-resistant HIV strain. To minimize such problems, it was recommended that HAART initiation in the United States be delayed until those affected at least reach the third stage of the disease.

Moreover, serious side effects are a potential outcome of treatment with highly active antiretroviral drugs. Equally important are concerns that studies regarding the long-term impact of these drugs on the quality of life for those under therapy are still lacking. In that regard, it appeared logical to delay HAART initiation until later stages of the disease, except for expectant mothers who need prevention from passing on the virus to the newborn during childbirth.

Ugandan HAART-providing centers and those of the United States also take different treatment approaches. U.S. centers such as 360: PCC take a holistic approach to treatment in which they provide comprehensive HIV/AIDS care to clients (360: PCC, 2008). Some of the services provided by U.S. HAART-providing centers include diagnostic tests; provision of medical care and medication, such as HIV drugs and laboratory and radiology services; medication services; outpatient surgical services; pain management; mental health counseling and treatment; and physical therapy and counseling; as well as comprehensive assessment and medical treatment for HIV and associated complications. Unlike those in Uganda, U.S. HAART-providing centers also offer social services that include referrals for assistance with community mental health, social support, housing assistance, disability services, nutrition, transportation, psychiatric care, health insurance, and home health care coordination (360: PCC, 2008; ASNT, 2007; Northwestern Memorial Hospital, 2008).

Although the Ugandan centers are designed to take a holistic approach to treatment—and despite the fact that they provide services such as free provision of anti-HIV drugs, tuberculosis treatment, and counseling—Ugandan centers cannot provide all needed services to clients because of financial constraints. For example, some of the opportunistic illnesses characteristic of individuals with advanced HIV (for instance, malignancies and shingles) are manifested in severe pain, but Ugandan centers can provide for neither their free treatment nor palliative care (USDS, 2007). All clients on HAART also need and are required by health care providers to access good nutrition (Food and Agriculture Organization [FAO], 2002). However, although the majority of individuals under therapy in Uganda cannot afford good nutrition, Ugandan centers cannot provide them with dietary supplements, as is the case in the United States (WHO, 2008b). Additionally, centers in Uganda do not possess laboratory equipment for effective diagnostic tests, such as those required for the CD4 cell count and viral load. The cost for these services is usually so high that those affected cannot afford them. These services are generally carried out by other organizations not affiliated with free HAART-providing centers and usually at a cost.

Despite their differences, Uganda's and the United States' HAART-providing centers also show some similarities. For instance, because HIV disproportionately affects those at the bottom of the social stratification in all societies, many of the providing centers both in the United States and in Uganda are nongovernmental organizations that provide free or subsidized services within local communities to those in need who cannot afford them (U.S. Global AIDS Coordinator, 2008). Another similarity is that most of the HIV centers in both countries were founded in the late 1980s or early 1990s. This was partially due to a delay on the part of the U.S. government and the world community to address the AIDS phenomenon soon after the initial HIV diagnoses in 1981 (Bongaarts, 1996; Robbins, 2005; TASO, 2006). Studies blame this delay on the stigma that surrounded the disease and those affected, who were supposedly labeled as homosexuals, prostitutes, sinners, or social deviants. Nevertheless, these nongovernmental programs expanded over time in size and efficiency. For example, all three satellite centers under study in Uganda are part of somewhat large nongovernmental organizations established in the 1990s. One of these centers belongs to an organization that has grown over the years, currently operating 35 centers nationwide that provide HAART to about 35,000 individuals (Mugyenyi et al., 2006). Another center is part of a nongovernmental organization that has also grown in size since its inception, currently operating 11 centers around the nation with a total enrollment of approximately 63,000 clients, of which about 14,000 were on HAART in 2005 (TASO, 2002). Increasing access to HAART in Uganda generates interest in studying its effects on those under therapy.

SIGNIFICANCE OF THE STUDY

The investigation of HAART adherence behavior and its effect on those under therapy in Uganda is important, especially because provision of HAART in low-income nations—such as those in sub-Saharan Africa, where many of the affected individuals are poverty stricken and possess little or no formal education—may result in negative public health implications, including those resulting from suboptimal adherence, such as drug resistance. That is, although long-term effects are still unknown, it is well documented that since its introduction in the mid-1990s, HAART has enhanced the quality of life for those individuals who adhere to treatment regimens (Wilson et al., 2002). However, some studies reveal that poor medication adherence may lead to progression of the disease and enhance its severity (Berg, Michelson, & Safren, 2007). For example, Altice, *Maru, Bruce, Springer, and Friedland* (2007) found that drug users in the United States have not had favorable outcomes from HAART partially as a result of poor adherence.

Some of the reasons individuals fail to adhere to medication regimens may be because prescription drugs are costly and individuals may be required to take medications on a full stomach. This raises concerns because most individuals in low-income nations live below the international poverty line and may not be able to afford food. For example, it is estimated that 852 million individuals around the world suffer from chronic hunger, of which 843 million live in developing nations where the majority of individuals makes less than one U.S. dollar a day (World Bank, 2011). Comparing the 2009 World Bank's GNI per capita statistical figures for low- and high-income nations, Uganda's GNI was $460 and that of Zimbabwe was only $360. In contrast, the United States' GNI was $46,360, that of Japan was $38,080, and that of the United Kingdom was $41,370 (World Bank, 2011). If the majority of those under therapy have insufficient access to food, taking medication on an empty stomach may cause nausea, which in turn may hinder individuals' ability to take medication as required and thus lead to the development of drug-resistant HIV. Because studies in this area are scarce, this study expands this very limited knowledge, and it may provide additional information on patterns of adherence and the quality of life for those under treatment in resource-constrained nations.

Additionally, increasing access to HAART in resource-constrained nations also raises the necessity for new knowledge pertaining to individual sexual behavior for those under therapy. Because HIV is an infectious yet chronic illness that currently has no cure, prevention—such as the regular use of condoms, having only one sex partner, or abstinence from sex—remains the best strategy in the control of the disease. In exploring the effect of HAART on sexual behavior of those under therapy, this study may augment existing knowledge pertaining to this area in resource-constrained nations. Of supreme importance, this study may assist in the formulation of strategies and policies that could enhance the effect of HAART and the quality of life for those with HIV/AIDS in developing nations such as Uganda.

Key Definitions

The following terms and concepts will be used in this study:

1. Anti-HIV drugs: Anti-HIV drugs refer to antiretroviral drugs.
2. Antiretroviral drugs (ARVs): Antiretroviral drugs refer to a class of therapeutic agents used to inhibit or slow the replication of retroviruses such as HIV. In so doing, ARVs slow the growth of

the virus and hence progression of the disease from HIV to AIDS (Last, 2007). ARV drugs include reverse transcriptase inhibitors and the PIs (*Concise Medical Dictionary*, 2008).

3. HAART: HAART is an abbreviation for highly active antiretroviral therapy. In this study, HAART refers to aggressive ARV drug treatment regimens used to suppress HIV viral replication and the promotion of HIV healthy living behaviors, such as good nutrition and safe sex practices—abstinence from sex if possible, using condoms during sexual intercourse, or having only one sex partner. The usual HAART regimen combines three or more different drugs that may include two NRTIs and a PI, two NRTIs and an NNRTI, or other such combinations.
4. HAART adherence: HAART adherence in this study is defined as how closely one follows a prescribed medication regimen as well as lifestyle recommendations. Adherence in this study is operationally defined by responses to questions that measure compliance to the providers' treatment regimens.
5. HIV healthy lifestyle recommendations: HIV healthy lifestyle recommendations in this study refer to abstinence from sex, or having sex with one partner, or always using a condom; abstinence from alcohol; and maintaining good nutrition.
6. Perceived quality of life: Perceived quality of life is defined as the individual's perception of his or her physical and psychological well-being. Perceived quality of life in this study is operationally defined by responses to self-reported measures pertaining to how an individual perceives his or her physical and psychological health.

Chapter 2

Treating HIV/AIDS

Highly Active Antiretroviral Therapy and Quality of Life

HIV is treated with antiretroviral drugs. These drugs do not cure but rather control the virus by hindering its rapid replication and hence the destruction of CD4 cells. The initial days of HIV treatment utilized one antiretroviral drug, such as AZT, and treatment was basically referred to as antiretroviral therapy (ART). However, because of the high potential to develop drug-resistant HIV, the invention of additional compounds led to what may be referred to as a medical breakthrough in 1996, when it was discovered that a more effective way to repress HIV replication required a combination of various types of anti-HIV drugs, a treatment known as highly active antiretroviral therapy (HAART). Irrefutably, since its implementation HAART has led to clinical improvements in the health of those infected with HIV. Because of these anti-HIV drugs, AIDS has been downgraded from what was initially perceived as an automatic death sentence to a complex but controllable chronic illness.

Statistically, soon after HAART's introduction, the HIV incidence declined by 38% and the AIDS mortality rate dropped by 63% worldwide (Berg et al., 2007; Garcia & Cote, 2003; Harrigan et al., 2005; Morbidity and Mortality Weekly Report, 2003).

Studies—especially those conducted in developed nations—reveal that morbidity from HIV opportunistic infections has almost been eliminated by HAART, which has contributed to improved health and increased longevity for those living with the virus (Gao et al., 2000; Laing & Hodgkin, 2006; Palella et al., 1998). For example, Lohse, Hansen, Gerstoft, and Obel (2007) called HAART a medical success that boosts the CD4 cell count, eventually improving the physical and psychological health for those under treatment. Mannheimer et al. (2005) also noted immunological and virological gains for those under HAART. Rowell and Shippy (2004) further revealed improvements in the mental health, social function, and overall quality of life among study participants under HAART. Studies pertaining to the impact of HAART on the quality of life for those infected with the virus in developing countries remain scarce, but the few extant studies reveal somewhat similar findings as those noted previously. For example, statistics reveal a reduction in the AIDS mortality rate in Botswana attributed to 3 years of effective treatment with highly active antiretroviral drugs (WHO, 2008a). In a study conducted in South Africa, Jelsma, Maclean, Hughes, Tinese, and Darder (2005) found improvement in the quality of life and increase in the survival rate for individuals treated with anti-HIV drugs after they were diagnosed with AIDS. Such clinical improvements in health for those under HAART, if accessible, continue to inspire hope for a cure among those with HIV/AIDS worldwide.

Access to Highly Active Antiretroviral Drugs

As discussed previously, the introduction of HAART was a medical breakthrough in the treatment of HIV. However, because of the high cost of anti-HIV drugs, the majority of those who need treatment especially in resource-limited regions cannot access these drugs without financial assistance (Laing & Hodgkin, 2006; UNAIDS, 2006c). Therefore, the millennium began with the international community's mobilization efforts to provide and increase HAART access in these regions (UNAIDS, 2006a; WHO, 2006b). For example, the U.S.-based PEPFAR, which was formulated in 2003, had a goal to provide treatment to about 2 million individuals affected by HIV/AIDS worldwide within 5 years (USDS, 2004). PEPFAR's initial plan was to spend approximately $15 billion primarily in low-income nations chosen based on U.S. political views to fight HIV/AIDS, tuberculosis, and malaria; this expenditure was increased to about $48 billion in 2008 by President Obama to fund the same plan for an additional 5 years (UNAIDS, 2010a). From 2003 to 2010, the number of individuals receiving antiretroviral drugs through PEPFAR specifically in sub-Saharan Africa increased from 50,000 to about 3.2 million (USDS, 2011). Similar to the efforts of the United States, WHO also introduced a "3 by 5" initiative in 2003 with an objective to "provide access to HAART to 3 million people in developing countries by 2005" (UNAIDS, 2006a; WHO, 2006a). The United Nations member states scaled up these initiatives with a goal for everyone affected by the virus to access HAART by 2010 (WHO, 2006b). Despite the fact that the United Nations fell short of its 2010 goal, with only about 42% of those in need receiving HAART by the end of 2008, the international community continues to assist low-income nations in accessing anti-HIV drugs. Among those living up to this mission, the Global Fund was the largest multilateral organization contributor in 2009. The United States through PEPFAR was the largest single donor nation in the fight against HIV/AIDS during the same year, followed by the United Kingdom through the Department for International Development (DFID) (UNAIDS, 2010b). Some of the other nations helping poor nations access anti-HIV drugs include France, Sweden, Canada, Germany, Ireland, the Netherlands, Italy, Australia, Japan, Norway, and Denmark. There is no doubt that the effort to scale up HAART in low-income nations is beneficial. However, with it comes public health concerns, such as those springing from adherence failure (the potential for the development of drug-resistant HIV), and hence treatment failure and increase in the infection rate, all of which undermine the international community's efforts to control HIV (Munro, Lewin, Swart, & Volmink, 2007; Redding, Rossi, Rossi, Velicer, & Prochaska, 2000).

Defining HAART and Medication Adherence

Before discussing public health implications of adherence failure and influential adherence factors, it is necessary to define medication and HAART adherence and understand its importance. HAART adherence in this study refers to medication adherence as well as following health providers' lifestyle recommendations that are crucial to the control of HIV infection. These recommendations include the execution of lifestyle changes such as maintaining good nutrition, refraining from alcohol, and engagement in safe sex practices; the last strategy is known as ABC, where A stands for abstinence until marriage, B for being faithful to one sex partner, and C for using a condom regularly if all of the previous are not possible (FAO, 2002; Schmitt & Mehta, 2002; WHO, 2003a; WHO, 2009a). In contrast, there is no standardized definition of medication adherence. However, researchers often refer to medication adherence as the extent to which patients take medication exactly as prescribed by health care providers in terms of dosing, frequency, and timing—a definition adopted in this study (Machtinger & Bangsberg, 2008; Park & Mayhorn, 1996; Weinberg & Friedland, 1998).

Medication Adherence Among Chronically Ill Patients

Researchers agree that effective treatment of HIV requires about 95% or higher medication adherence, which is especially difficult to achieve when treatment is long-term, as is the case for HIV, currently considered a chronic illness (Garcia & Cote, 2003; Hammer et al., 2006; Mannheimer, Friedland, Matts, Child, & Chesney, 2002). Research is unclear about how to measure 95% adherence. However, Machtinger and Bangsberg (2008) indicated that 95% adherence is attainable by not missing fewer than three doses in a month. Unfortunately, although adherence studies remain scarce, a few scholars have revealed that suboptimal adherence to HAART is common in all groups of treated individuals (Machtinger & Bangsberg, 2008; Munro et al., 2007). In Harrigan et al.'s

(2005) study conducted in Canada, about 43% of individuals on HAART had an adherence level of less than 95%. In a study conducted in Spain, Carballo et al. (2004) found that 44% of the 235 participants on HAART had less than a 95% adherence level. Various scholars indicate different adherence rates in the United States, but average adherence is estimated at 70% (DiMatteo, Giordani, Lepper, & Crogham, 2002; Machtinger & Bangsberg, 2008). A few studies conducted in sub-Saharan Africa also reveal various HAART adherence levels. For example, Hardon et al. (2007) reviewed six quantitative studies in Africa and found that 65% to 99% individuals on HAART showed an adherence level of 95%. In another study of 514 HAART clients interviewed in Botswana, only 23% of individuals indicated a dosage adherence level of less than 95% (WHO, 2008b). The same study also found that as many as 79% of the 207 patients interviewed in Tanzania were below the critical adherence level (WHO, 2008b). Research further reveals that even when individuals do not miss a dose, they may fail to take medication at the exact appointed time (Williams & Friedland, 1997). For example, Melbourne et al. (1999) found that 50% of study participants with a 90% dosing adherence level took medication not at the exact time but within two or more hours after the appointed time. Failure to take medication at the exact time is almost as detrimental to public health as missing doses, especially in reference to the development of drug-resistant HIV. Following are public concerns of adherence failure.

Public Health Implications of Adherence Failure

Medication Adherence and Drug-Resistant HIV

There is a strong correlation between intermittent medication dosing and causation of drug-resistant HIV, which is a menace to public health. Drug-resistant HIV leads to treatment failure because it cannot respond to anti-HIV drugs, yet it may be transmissible. In explaining the formation of drug-resistant HIV, it is important to understand that the purpose of treating HIV with highly active antiretroviral drugs is not to cure but to suppress the virus or halt its replication (Machtinger & Bangsberg,

2008; Mills et al., 2006; UNAIDS, 2006a; WHO, 2006a). Effective suppression of HIV requires a certain concentration level of combination anti-HIV drugs in the blood system to which the viral replication is exposed, a level that is maintained with 95% and higher medication adherence as mentioned earlier (Descamps et al., 2000; Hogg et al., 2002; Laing & Hodgkin, 2006; Lucas, 2005; Machtinger & Bangsberg, 2008; Paterson et. al., 2000). Less than 95% adherence causes drug-resistant HIV because drugs are continuously excreted from the body through the digestive system, kidneys, and liver such that if not replaced as recommended, the drug concentration level is diluted below HIV repression capacity through food and water intake, giving the virus a chance to reshape. The process by which HIV changes shape is referred to as viral mutation, and it is more likely to occur when the viral load is high than when it is low (Laing & Hodgkin, 2006). The reshaped HIV is referred to as the drug-resistant strain because it makes drugs less effective at controlling it (Weinberg & Friedland, 1998; Wensing & Boucher, 2003). As the new drug-resistant virus makes copies of itself, resistance to a specific drug also increases until the drug becomes completely ineffective in controlling the HIV replication process, thus creating a need for a new combination drug that can effectively suppress the reshaped HIV (GlaxoSmithKline, 2008; Laing & Hodgkin, 2006; Weinberg & Friedland, 1998). Detrimental to public health is the fact that resistance to one drug is frequently associated with cross-resistance to other members of the same class of drugs, which limits future treatment options, specifically for those infected with the new HIV strain (Deeks et al., 2003; GlaxoSmithKline, 2008; Hogg et al., 2002).

Another public health concern in reference to drug resistance is treatment failure. That is, the purpose of anti-HIV drugs is to suppress HIV replication to a point at which it is undetectable in the blood system. However, when the virus changes shape, it begins to rapidly replicate itself in resistance to drug detection, thus increasing the HIV viral load in the blood system, which indicates treatment failure (Descamps et al., 2000; Mills et al., 2006). This is somewhat supported in the literature, as in Harrigan et al.'s (2005) study conducted in Canada, which revealed that HIV-resistant strains were more likely to occur in individuals whose plasma showed a low concentration of antiretroviral drugs as compared to those with high concentration levels. Bangsberg, Kroetz, and Deeks's (2007) study conducted in San Francisco also found that the viral load doubles for each 10% decrease in adherence. Increase in the viral load leads to increase in the rapid destruction of CD4 cells and hence disease progression from HIV to AIDS (Hogg et al., 2002; Machtinger & Bangsberg, 2008; Vanhove, Schapiro, Winters, Merigan, & Blaschke, 1996). For example, Machtinger and Bangsberg (2008) affirmed that suboptimal medication adherence is the second strongest predictor of progression from HIV to AIDS and death, after CD4 cell count. Likewise, in Kitahata et al.'s (2004) study, patients with low adherence had more than five times the risk of disease progression as compared to patients with moderate to high adherence levels. Hogg et al.'s (2002) study also correlated anti-HIV drug adherence rates to viral suppression and disease progression. Failure to effectively suppress HIV replication partially resulting from adherence failure undermines public health efforts to control the virus.

Additionally, public health is threatened with the fact that multi-drug-resistant viruses may be transmissible (Hogg et al., 2002; Weinberg & Friedland, 1998; Wensing & Boucher, 2003; Wilson et al., 2002). For example, although it is unclear if transmitted drug-resistant HIV was the result of adherence failure, very high rates of drug-resistant HIV strains were found in recently infected individuals in a study of 225 untreated patients infected with HIV, a study conducted at a public hospital in San Francisco between 1996 and 2001 (Grant et al., 2002). If drug-resistant HIV is transmissible, public health may be threatened with a new HIV strain whose infection rate may rapidly increase, especially in conducive environments such as those of sub-Saharan Africa that lack effective disease control mechanisms, such as health education and surveillance. Worse still is the fact that, despite potential increase in the incidence of a resistant HIV strain within a given community, available anti-HIV drugs to treat those affected may be unavailable. It is noteworthy that public health is concerned with not only clinical immunological gains that follow medication adherence but also sociological implications of HAART adherence as discussed later.

Adherence to Safe Sexual Practices

Individuals under HAART are advised to engage in safe sex practices because the purpose of HAART is to control HIV, not only in terms of treatment but also of the infection rate. Failure to adhere to safe sex practices is of public health concern because of the potential of increasing the HIV infection rate especially in developing countries such as those in sub-Saharan Africa, where the major HIV transmission mode is heterosexual intercourse (American Public Health Association [APHA], 2004; Essex & Mboup, 2002; USDS, 2007; U.S. Global AIDS Coordinator, 2008; Weinberg & Friedland, 1998; Wensing & Boucher, 2003). That is, as mentioned earlier, highly active antiretroviral drugs do not cure HIV but suppress the retrovirus or inhibit its replication to a point where HIV may be undetectable in the blood system (Berg et al., 2007; Hammer et al., 2006; Laing & Hodgkin, 2006; Mocroft et al., 2007). Important to note is the fact that some studies reveal that even when the viral load cannot be detected, memory T-lymphocytes that possess replication-competent HIV remain present in a resistant state and may stay in that form for decades (Deeks et al., 2003; Hammer et al., 2006; Siliciano, 2000). This means that the virus can still be passed on regardless of a negative HIV test. Although information on the degree of transmissibility of HIV from individuals with an undetectable viral load does not exist, replication-competent HIV from secretions of patients on HAART who have undetectable viral loads and the transmission of HIV—including drug-resistant strains—from HAART participants to uninfected patients have been documented in developed nations (APHA, 2004; Weinberg & Friedland, 1998; Wensing & Boucher, 2003). It is for such reasons that effective implementation of HAART recommends safe sex practices for those under therapy.

Adherence to Good Nutrition

Another recommendation for individuals on HAART is good nutrition. Although good nutrition cannot suppress or cure HIV, HAART health care providers recommend it because it contributes to a better overall quality of life. For example, good nutrition may boost the function of the immune system, assist in the replacement or repair of bodily tissues and cells, help maintain the right body temperature, and assist carrying out chemical processes such as food digestion, all of which may maximize the effectiveness of HAART (FAO, 2002; San Francisco AIDS Foundation [SFAF], 2007). Good nutrition may also assist in managing certain health conditions common among individuals suffering from AIDS, such as diarrhea or vomiting, which may in turn reinforce the effectiveness of antiretroviral drug treatment (Brownell & Cohen, 1995; FAO, 2002). For example, diarrhea is an opportunistic illness commonly experienced by individuals with HIV/AIDS, and it may also be induced as a side effect of HAART. Diarrhea leads to loss of water and minerals from the body, which vomiting may elevate, a loss that may be replenished by good nutrition (Brownell & Cohen, 1995). Unfortunately, as discussed before, many of those on HAART—especially in low-income nations, most of whom are usually positioned at the bottom of the social stratification system—fail to adhere to health providers' advice in reference to good nutrition, partially because they cannot afford a good diet. Another influential factor for failure to comply with good nutrition recommendations is side effects. According to the literature, side effects such as nausea, vomiting, or diarrhea may partially hinder adherence to good nutrition because these conditions can complicate food intake—for instance, altering the taste of food or causing one to lose one's appetite (Hardon et al., 2007; Moyer et al., 1999; SFAF, 2007).

Adherence to Sobriety

Individuals on HAART are also recommended to refrain from mind-altering drugs including alcohol for several reasons. First, alcohol is a chemical that may interfere with drug compounds, which in turn may interfere with the effectiveness of antiretroviral drugs. Second, alcohol may be associated with adherence failure partially because of its potential to cause patients to forget to take medication as required (FAO, 2002; Hardon et al., 2006; Haubrich et al., 1999; Moatti et al., 2000).

For example, in Paterson et al.'s (2000) study, patients' use of alcohol was strongly associated with adherence levels of less than 95%. In a study conducted in the United States, Halkitis, Palamar, and Mukherjee (2008) also linked mind-altering drug use to poor medication adherence. Additionally, alcohol use may foster engagement in risky sexual behavior such as high-risk unplanned or casual sexual intercourse and failure to remember to use a condom. Equally important is the fact that alcohol intake has the potential to reduce food appetite, which may then foster adherence failure because some medications must be taken on a full stomach. As indicated earlier, HAART adherence failure minimizes public health efforts to control HIV as well as to improve the quality of life for those under therapy. Therefore, before finding solutions to adherence failure, it is important to understand causes for adherence failure.

Factors Influencing Adherence

HAART adherence failure may be attributed to illness and medication representation; complex treatment regimens in reference to frequency, dosing, timing, and dietary expectations; psychosocial factors such as depression, social support, doctor-patient relationships, clinical setting, and demographic characteristics; and other factors, such as mind-altering drug use and stigma, as elaborated in the following sections (Hardon et al., 2007; Munro et al., 2007).

Medication Representation

One of the major influential factors for adherence failure is medication representation. Medication representation refers to beliefs pertaining to the effect of specific medications on a particular illness, which may be formulated based on an individual's past experiences and which may shape that individual's perception of a particular drug and its effects on a specific illness (Park & Mayhorn, 1996). For instance, numerous studies agree that if patients know the importance of the medication they are taking, they are more likely to remember taking it, as opposed to those who have doubts about the same medication (Leventhal & Cameron,

1987; Williams & Friedland, 1997). As Park and Mayhorn (1996) put it, individuals who believe medications are effective in controlling an illness that interferes substantially with everyday life are more likely to adhere to medication regimens. Examples of such illnesses (in reference to AIDS-related conditions) might include itching, red eyes, skin rash, migraine headache, herpes zoster, arthritis, and shingles, to name only a few.

Side Effects

Correspondingly, perception of medication as the source of undesirable side effects also has an impact on adherence (Berg et al., 2007; Giles & Brennan, 2001; Hardon et al., 2007; Kalichman et al., 2001; Samet et al., 1992). As discussed before, all highly active antiretroviral drugs have side effects that vary by drug, severity, individual, and interaction with other drugs including alcohol (McNicholl, 2007). Some of the side effects are severe or life threatening and may include liver problems, diabetes, high cholesterol, high levels of lactate in the blood, abnormal fat distribution, and decreased bone density (Laing & Hodgkin, 2006). According to Ammassari et al. (2001), side effects are frequent in HIV-positive individuals treated with HAART and occur in 29% to 36% of subjects, usually evidenced after 14 to 19 months of observation. Despite trust in the effectiveness of medication, antiretroviral drugs that generate side effects may lead to low levels of adherence. For example, a study conducted in Italy showed strong correlations between side effects such as anxiety, fatigue, abnormal fat accumulation, nausea, anorexia, and insomnia and adherence to HAART (Ammassari et al., 2001). In another study, conducted in India, Safren et al. (2005) also found that side effects were associated with irregular adherence behavior. A study of HAART adherence levels conducted in Uganda, Tanzania, and Botswana revealed somewhat similar results (Hardon et al., 2007).

Illness Representation

Furthermore, other scholars have argued that the more serious the disease, the higher adherence is; many serious illnesses result in unpleasant symptoms, discomfort, or pain that may materialize into constant sources of concern and anxiety, acting as reminders to take corrective measures (Gao et al., 2000; Park & Mayhorn, 1996; Williams & Friedland, 1997). Garcia and Cote (2003) also argued that how a patient perceives the seriousness of the disease and the degree to which he or she believes a given medication can control it affect adherence behavior. Illness representation and adherence association is important in resource-limited settings because one of the conditions for free HAART initiation, based on WHO's access guidelines, is experience with serious opportunistic illnesses such as tuberculosis, chronic diarrhea, wasting syndrome, prolonged fever, and PCP (Daniels, 2005; Laing & Hodgkin, 2006; Munro et al., 2007). A few studies associate prior history of opportunistic infections with HAART adherence (Gao et al., 2000; Singh et al., 1996).

Illness representation may influence not only medication adherence but also failure to comply with health providers' recommendations such as refraining from risky sexual behavior (Munro et al., 2007). A few studies conducted in high-income nations indicate that when some individuals on HAART learn that their viral load is undetectable or receive an improved prognosis, they may become less apprehensive or cautious about safe sex because of a false perception that they are no longer infectious. Findings about sexual behavior among individuals on HAART in that regard remain inconclusive. Some studies state that individuals who perceive themselves as not infectious if on HAART may engage in sexual practices with HIV risks, such as sexual intercourse with multiple partners or unprotected sex (Lohse et al., 2007; Remien et al., 2007; Schwartlander et al., 2001). This is a danger to public health because such individuals may be reinfected with a different strain of HIV or may even infect others, both of which undermine public health efforts to control the virus. Few studies that link risky sexual behavior to HAART in developing countries exist (Krishnan et al., 2007). In Bateganya et al.'s (2005) study, 35% of the 348 respondents on HAART in Uganda reported more than one sex partner. In a study conducted in India, a significant number of males on HAART did not utilize condoms (Krishnan et al., 2007). The same study also revealed that women on HAART expressed powerlessness to decide on safe sexual practices such as the use of condoms. In contrast, other studies, some of which are conducted in developed nations, reveal that individuals on HAART are less likely to engage in unprotected sex than those who are not under treatment (Crepaz, Hart, & Marks, 2004).

Complex Treatment Regimens

Another factor that has the potential to influence medication adherence behavior is a complex treatment regimen in terms of the number, smell, and size of pills; dosing schedules; and if medications are to be taken with or without food (Machtinger & Bangsberg, 2008; Mills et al., 2006; Moyer et al., 1999). That is, HAART regimens may require intake of multiple pills several times a day (Garcia & Cote, 2003; Moyer et al., 1999; Weidle, Malamb, Mwebaze, & Sozi, 2002; Williams & Friedland, 1997). Additionally, some pills may be significantly big in size and smell and taste unpleasant, which may cause an individual to refrain from taking medication as recommended. The smell, size, taste, and number of pills per given dose may be a problem especially where medication has to be taken for life, as is the case with anti-HIV medication. Numerous scholars agree that taking antiretroviral drugs several times a day, often taking multiple tablets per dose, is a challenge that influences medication-taking behavior (Bartlett, DeMasi, Quinn, Moxham, & Rousseau, 2001; Laing & Hodgkin, 2006; Machtinger & Bangsberg, 2008). This is also supported by Boyle's (2005) study of 219 patients in New York, which found that individuals whose medication-taking regimens were reduced to once daily showed higher adherence levels as compared to those with twice-daily regimens.

Dietary needs also influence adherence behavior. For example, some medications must be taken on a full stomach, which may affect medication-taking behavior especially in low-income countries, where food may be costly for those under therapy. For instance, a study conducted in Uganda revealed that people would stop taking medication because of a lack of food (WHO, 2008b). In a study conducted in South Africa, Abah et al. (2005) also found a link between access to food and adherence failure. Similarly, in Hardon et al.'s (2007) study, absence of food caused some participants on a twice-a-day dosing regimen to take their antiretroviral drugs only once a day. As discussed before, intermittent dosing is a danger to public health because it may result in treatment failure.

Depression

Clinical depression—feelings of hopelessness, fatigue, or social isolation—is common among individuals under HAART, yet it is highlighted in literature as an indicator of adherence (Ammassari et al., 2001; Cook, Grey, & Burke, 2004; DiMatteo et al., 2002; Farinpour, Miller, & Satz, 2003; Singh et al., 1996). For example, in a study conducted in the United States, Komiti et al. (2003) found that clinical depression affects about 20% of individuals living with HIV/AIDS. However, DiMatteo, Lepper, and Croghan's (2000) meta-analysis study showed that depressed people had three times the risk of low adherence behavior compared to those who were not depressed. In another study, conducted in Italy, Ammassari et al. (2001) also found a link between nonadherence and depression. Carballo et al. (2004) revealed somewhat similar results in a study conducted in Spain. Depression's potential effects on adherence failure may be partially attributed to loss of energy or feelings of hopelessness that may cause one to stay in bed and hence sleep through the dose.

Social Support

Furthermore, scholars highlight social support or the presence of other individuals in a household as an influential factor in adherence behavior (Machtinger & Bangsberg, 2008; Munro et al., 2007; Park & Mayhorn, 1996; Singh et al., 1999; WHO, 2008b; Williams & Friedland, 1997). For example, Holzemer et al. (1999) found that people living with HIV who lacked social support were less likely to adhere to medication regimens or health providers' advice as compared to those who had social support. Gordillo et al.'s (1999) study also revealed that individuals with social support are more likely to adhere to medication regimens than those without support. High medication adherence may be attributed to the fact that those with social support could be reminded by others to comply or reminded of the importance of adherence to health providers' recommendations, such as taking medication as required or avoiding risky sexual behavior. One of the contributing factors to lack of social support may be fear to disclose one's HIV serostatus. This fear may spring from the fact that HIV is stigmatized and disclosure may pose sociological implications, such as discrimination or abandonment by significant others. The literature links fear of stigmatization with failure to disclose one's serostatus and hence with lack of social support (Hardon et al., 2007). For instance, in a study conducted in South Africa, Abah et al. (2005) found that highly active antiretroviral drug users sometimes find this difficult to disclose to family members, which denies them access to adherence support.

Doctor-Patient Relationship

Numerous studies associate patient-provider relationship characteristics—such as provider support, patient's opinion of the provider's competence, and satisfaction and trust in staff—with adherence behavior (Machtinger & Bangsberg, 2008; Williams & Friedland, 1997). In Lucas, Chaisson, and Moore's (1999) study, high levels of medication adherence and compliance with provider lifestyle recommendations correlated with health provider support. Gordillo et al.'s (1999) study also found a strong association between HAART adherence and support from the health provider and, conversely, between missing doctor's appointments and lack of health provider support. As Park and Mayhorn (1996) put it, health provider support such as caring is crucial for adherence given challenging health experiences faced by individuals with HIV. Studies that link provider support and adherence to treatment in low-income countries remain scarce. In one of these studies, Hardon et al. (2007) found provider support for individuals on HAART in Tanzania poor, which was attributed to a heavy health provider workload. Individuals on HAART who are supported by health care providers may adhere to treatment recommendations because providers assist them in understanding the importance of treatment as well as in overcoming social-psychological obstacles to adherence, such as depression, fear of being seen in public taking anti-HIV medication, and so forth, which could be achieved through counseling.

Clinical Setting

Clinical setting features such as location of the facility, transportation to and from the clinic, childcare, waiting time, and pleasantness of the clinical environment have also been associated with adherence behavior (Machtinger & Bangsberg, 2008; Munro et al., 2007). In Uganda, for example, some HAART clients indicated that the distance to health facilities was a hindrance to adherence because they could not afford transportation to and from the clinic for prescription refills (WHO, 2008b). Hardon et al.'s (2007) study also found that although antiretroviral drugs are free, transportation costs prohibited individuals under therapy in East African countries from traveling to clinics to refill prescriptions. If individuals fail to refill prescriptions on a timely basis, they may be forced to skip taking medication in between refills.

Demographic Characteristics

Furthermore, a few scholars link adherence behavior to some of the sociodemographic factors, such as age and education (Garcia & Cote, 2003; Kalichman, Ramachandran, & Catz, 1999; Kerr, Weitkunat, & Moretti, 2005; Machtinger & Bangsberg, 2008; Weinberg & Friedland, 1998). For instance, Mannheimer et al. (2002) found a correlation between old age and better adherence levels. In Paterson et al.'s (2000) study, older patients were more likely to have 95% or greater adherence than the younger patients. Gordillo et al.'s (1999) study, conducted in Madrid between 1997 and 1998, also found that individuals above age 32 were more likely to adhere to medication as compared to their younger counterparts. Similarly, Halkitis et al.'s (2008) study in 2004 of 300 HIV-positive men that have sex with men in New York revealed that individuals over age 50 were more likely to adhere to highly active antiretroviral drugs than their younger counterparts. One of the reasons why older individuals may be more compliant with treatment regimens may be because better medication-taking experience may come with age. Older people may also have fewer daily interruptions than their younger counterparts, who are likely to still be engaged in the labor force or be busy with family activities. Illness representation as discussed previously could also be influential, whereby older individuals may be more cautious about their health as opposed to younger individuals.

Education is also associated with adherence. For instance, Carballo et al.'s (2004) study conducted in Spain found that individuals with higher education were more adherent to HAART than those who had no primary education. Similarly, Gordillo et al. (1999) found that individuals with low education had the lowest adherence rates as compared to those who had some college education. Studies that link low education to adherence failure lead to speculation that individuals on HAART in Africa, many of whom live in poverty and lack formal education, may fail to adhere to HAART, which could lead to the development and spread of drug-resistant HIV (Mills et al., 2006). One of the reasons why those without education may not comply with health providers' recommendations is financial constraints. That is, there is a strong correlation among education, occupation, and income, whereby the less educated are more likely to be at the bottom of the social stratification system. For instance, as indicated earlier, if lack of transport to the clinic for refills contributes to adherence failure, it is usually the uneducated who are more likely to lack the means to access medication on a timely basis because they cannot afford the transportation costs. In the same regard, the uneducated may also be less likely to afford food than the educated. Because some medication must be taken on a full stomach, lack of food may influence poor adherence.

Other Factors Influencing Adherence

HIV/AIDS stigma can also lead to poor adherence because affected individuals may feel insecure disclosing their HIV condition to fellow workers or significant others in fear of being rejected. For instance, in Hardon et al.'s (2007) study, participants indicated that disclosure had caused them to lose their jobs or to be abandoned by family and friends. Those who fear to disclose might also be afraid to take anti-HIV medication in public because it may be a sign to others that they have the virus. To avoid revealing their status, some people may skip taking medication while in public places such as work, or they may wait and take it late after they get to a confidential location. This argument is supported by Hardon et al.'s (2007) study, which found that fear of being seen by colleagues, family, or friends while taking HIV medication caused individuals to skip taking medication as prescribed.

Moreover, mind-altering drugs including alcohol may contribute to adherence failure in that one may forget to take medication as required, or alcohol may make one sleep through the dose. Some individuals merely forget to take medication at the required time. Others who fail to carry medication with them at all times may also skip taking medication, for instance, when they are traveling. Still others may skip taking medication in between refills because employers do not give them time off to travel to the clinic to refill prescriptions (Kalichman et al., 2001).

Social Theories and Adherence Behavior

Sick Role Theory

Talcott Parsons (1951) in his sick role theory perceived illness as an anomaly to the human body that must be rectified partially by the ill person, who is expected to comply with sick role normative behavior. Parsons's argument is that the sick are blameless because illness is beyond their control. However, they are obligated to choose better health by seeking and complying with treatment regimens, whereas failure to do so qualifies them as deviants (Parsons, 1951). In addition, illness should not be self-inflicted. In application of the sick role theory to HAART adherence, good health should be in the self-interest of those under therapy, who are obligated by society to choose health-promoting behaviors such as practicing medication adherence and HIV-risk-free sexual behavior, refraining from mind-altering drug use including alcohol, and adhering to good nutrition as advised by health professionals (Coreil, Bryant, & Henderson, 2001). Individuals who fail to do so are accountable for their actions. Of concern to researchers is the question of why individuals fail to adhere to sick role behavior, such as complying with health providers' recommendations. Psychosocial and public health theories are often drawn on to answer this question.

However, before proceeding, it is important to understand that none of the existing theories fully explain HAART adherence failure especially in developing nations, probably because these theories were initially formulated to explain health behavior in developed nations. Even the sick role theory is limited because it does not consider social contexts in which sick role obligations may be beyond the control of the sick person, like circumstances where gender power imbalances mean that females may not have power to negotiate safe sex with their partners. Nevertheless, HAART adherence behavior in resource-constrained nations may be best understood through the integration of various existing theoretical paradigms, such as the social support theory and theories that take a cognitive approach—the health belief model (HBM), the social cognitive theory (SCT), and the theory of reasoned action (TRA)/theory of planned behavior (TPB) (Redding et al., 2000). Additionally, the rational choice theory (RCT), the theory of gender power, the communication-motivational theory, and the communication theory can also be drawn on to explain HAART adherence behavior, especially in resource-limited settings such as those in sub-Saharan Africa.

Social Support Model

Emile Durkheim was the first sociologist to explain health behavior by linking social support and social integration. The theory of social support is mentioned in numerous studies that attempt to predict health behavior (Durkheim, 1897/1951). Durkheim explored differing suicide rates among Catholics and Protestants in the late 1880s in Europe and found that suicide rates were higher among affluent Protestants as compared to less affluent Catholics; he theorized that affluent Protestants were more suicidal than the less affluent Catholics because the Protestants were more individualistic and less socially integrated in the community and the less affluent Catholics experienced a higher degree of community social integration. Although Durkheim's study is limited (partially because of its highly descriptive nature and the population under study), the literature shows substantial evidence accumulated from numerous qualitative and quantitative studies that link heath outcomes such as complying with providers' health recommendations to social support. Scholars agree that affectionate, loving relationships from friends and kin usually have the potential to increase a sense of self-efficacy or modify an individual's feelings, thoughts, or behavior (Redding et al., 2000). For example, loving relationships may strengthen coping skills for those on HAART by helping them deal with adherence in the midst of manifestations of side effects as well as by building their self-efficacy. For example, in Cobbs' (1976) study, social support from family, friends, and health care providers was a significant indicator of medication adherence.

Health Belief Model

Another theory that may be utilized in the explanation of health behavior is the health belief model, formulated in the 1950s by social psychologists (Holwerda, 2000; MSUCARES, 2001). According to the HBM, health behavioral change occurs after one makes rational assessments in terms of benefits and barriers to an action (Munro et al., 2007). The driving forces behind adherence behavior according to scholars who utilize this theory are perceived susceptibility, perceived seriousness, perceived benefits, and perceived barriers, forces that are often influenced by demographic and sociopsychological variables (WHO, 2003a). In applying this theory to HAART, individuals are more likely to take medications as prescribed and to comply with health providers' lifestyle recommendations if they perceive their health status to be serious, perceive the progression of HIV/AIDS as a threat, perceive benefits such as improved quality of life, are not overwhelmed by costs such as side effects from anti-HIV medications, and are confident they can adhere to health providers' recommendations successfully (Haisch & Hornung, 2005; Holwerda, 2000; MSUCARES, 2001).

Social Cognitive Theory

Another theory that can explain HAART adherence behavior and that is widely applied to health behaviors, specifically in reference to unhealthy lifestyles such as poor diet, is Bandura's social cognitive theory (Bandura, 2002). From the perspective of the SCT, health behavior may change based on the following: knowledge of health benefits, negative or positive expected outcome, risks, perceived facilitators or barriers, and self-efficacy whereby self-efficacy means belief in the accomplishment of a specific action necessary to achieve a given outcome (Bandura, 2002; Redding et al., 2000). For example, individuals are more likely to adhere to HAART if they are confident they have the power to take their medications as prescribed, believe they have the power to change their quality of life, believe highly active antiretroviral drugs will do more good than harm, and have few barriers such as those relating to side effects (Luszczynska & Sutton, 2005; Munro et al., 2007). When Keller, Fleury, Gregor-Holt, and Thompson (1999) conducted a 27-study systematic review that utilized SCT in the 1990s to explore the association between self-efficacy and physical activity, they concluded that SCT is a good indicator of physical activity.

Theories of Reasoned Action

Additionally, the theory of reasoned action may also be used to explain health behaviors. This theory is related to the theory of planned behavior, which is an extension of the TRA that was formulated to address limitations of the TRA by accommodating environmental control predictors of health behavior not addressed by the TRA (Munro et al., 2007; Redding et al., 2000). Based on the TRA, behavior is under volitional control and is determined by one's level of intention, perception, and outcome and significant others' opinions in relation to a particular behavior (Luszczynska & Sutton, 2005; MSUCARES, 2001; Redding et al., 2000). Based on this theory, intention is influenced by attitudes or values, self-efficacy, and subjective norms (MSUCARES, 2001). In that regard, individuals who conceptualize attitudes into values are more likely to adhere. For example, patients who feel HAART adherence leads to a better quality of life are more likely to adhere than those who believe otherwise (Redding et al., 2000). In addition, HAART adherence may be partially determined by one's thoughts of how significant others feel about adherence. In other words, individuals who feel significant others expect them to adhere to HAART are more likely to do so because of the social pressure exerted on them (MSUCARES, 2001).

Rational Choice Theory

Although missing from health behavior literature, RCT may also partially explain HAART adherence. Based on this theory, behavior results from a rational decision-making process through a careful evaluation of the costs and benefits that follow a particular act whereby the goal is to maximize benefits while minimizing costs (Kerr et al., 2005). In the case of HAART adherence, costs may refer to physical pain from disease progression. Benefits may pertain to the temporary relief from side effects manifested through suboptimal adherence or to peace of mind that may result from avoiding stigmatization if others learn that an individual is taking HIV medications (Liska & Messner, 1999). For example, a client on HAART who fails to adhere to medication regimens because of side effects may choose the instant reward of avoiding the pain manifested in these side effects in exchange for future consequences of disease progression. The choice of immediate gratification and risky health behavior such as intermittent medication intake is a menace to society because it does not only cost the individual; it will be a cost to society at a later date if, for instance, intermittent medication adherence causes resistant HIV and it spreads among members of a given community.

Theory of Gender Power

Robert Connell's emerging theory of gender power formulated in 1987—which focuses on the influence of social and cultural gender inequalities on female health—cannot be undermined, especially in the explanation of HAART adherence behavior in low-income settings (Connell, 1987; Crosby, Kegler, & DiClemente, 2002; Wingood & DiClemente, 2000).

Several researchers apply this theory in the examination of risky sexual behaviors in societies that portray gender power imbalances, such as those where cultural values deny females power to choose safe sex or to control the sexual behavior of their male counterparts (as with polygamy) (Buve et al., 2002). For example, in his application of this theory to a study of Latino females in Massachusetts, Pulerwitz, Amaro, De Jong, Gortmaker, and Rudd (2002) found that females who portrayed lower levels of relationship power were about five times less likely than those with higher levels of relationship power to use condoms. Sa and Larsen (2006) also found a strong association between gender inequalities and condom use among women in Tanzania. Inability of females to choose safe sex puts them at risk of acquiring sexually transmitted illnesses.

Protection-Motivation Theory

The protection motivation theory (PMT) may also be used to explain adherence behavior. This theory asserts that changes in behavior result from how an individual perceives the degree of severity of a threat, the degree of certainty that the threat will materialize, the efficacy of recommended preventive behavior, and the perceived self-efficacy or the level of self-confidence in one's ability to undertake the recommended preventive behavior (Rogers, 1975). In application of this theory to HAART adherence, individuals who perceive HIV progression to AIDS as a threat resulting from suboptimal adherence, who are certain that a drug-resistant HIV will evolve if they fail to adhere to medication regimens, who believe that antiretroviral drugs are effective, and who believe they have the power to adhere to health providers' recommendations are more likely to comply to medication regimens (Munro et al., 2007; Prentice-Dunn & Rogers, 1986).

Communication Perspective Theoretical Approach

Although rarely utilized, the communication perspective theoretical approach (CPT) may also help understand adherence behavior (Munro et al., 2007). Communication perspective theoretical analysts emphasize the importance of the patient–health provider relationship in influencing health behavior (WHO, 2003b). Talcott Parsons was one of the first social theorists to stress the importance of a supportive doctor-patient relationship in the effective treatment of the sick. In his sick role theory formulated in the 1950s, Parsons characterized the doctor's role in response to the sick as beneficent, which is essential for positive treatment outcomes (Parsons, 1951). Research reveals that individuals with skilled health providers who support and effectively communicate to clients in a comprehensible manner are more likely to adhere to HAART as compared to those without such providers (WHO, 2003b).

LIMITATIONS OF EXISTING THEORIES

Nevertheless, although none of the existing theories may fully explain adherence behavior, significant theoretical contributions may be drawn on to explain this phenomenon. The sick role theory, RCT, PMT, and cognitive theories such as HBM, TRA, and SCT tend to blame the individual; they also overlook behavior that is often constrained by external environmental controls, such as religious and cultural beliefs. For example, some behaviors—for instance, engagement in sex with multiple partners—may be rooted in cultural beliefs beyond individual control, such as those that value procreation and polygamy. Based on such beliefs, many African cultures encourage men to have several wives, which increases the risk of HIV infection within a given community. Females are also usually expected to submit to males in such a way that they are even denied the power to make decisions to engage in safe sexual practices. Other behavior may be rooted in society, where there are consequences of HIV/AIDS stigmatization: for instance, where one skips taking medication or takes medication late from fear of being seen taking anti-HIV drugs in public places, such as work. Or behavior may be influenced by financial constraints—skipping taking medication that is recommended to be taken on a full stomach in cases where the individual cannot afford food (Becker, 1985; Munro et al., 2007). Another behavior that existing theories may fail to address is engagement in sex for material gain, which is common in low-income nations. This behavior results from financial need.

To address limitations of one of these theories, Icez Azjen later formulated the theory of planned behavior, which extends the TRA to include behavior rooted in social contexts of which individuals have no control. However, even with Ajzen's extension of the TRA, the TPB remains limited because it fails to fully explain HAART adherence behavior. For example, in a meta-analysis of 24 studies conducted in Australia, the United States, Canada, and the Netherlands that employed the TPB to predict intention and health behavior such as exercise and cessation of smoking, Hardeman et al. (2002) found that variance in intention could be predicted in only 50% of the studies, and behavioral change was only explained in 33% of the studies.

Furthermore, even using the HBM, which is one of the most widely utilized theories, some studies often leave a large percentage of unexplained variance in health behavior, and others reveal inconclusive results (Haisch & Hornung, 2005; Munro et al., 2007; Redding et al., 2000; Rosenstock, 1974). For instance, Petosa and Jackson's (1991) study of safe sex indicators among adolescents in South Carolina found that the HBM could only explain 43% of the variance in safe sex among the 7th-grade students, 27% among 9th-grade students, and 17% of the variance among the 11th-grade students. Holwerda's (2000) study also found a positive correlation between perceived barriers and perceived susceptibility with self breast examination, but the correlation was insignificant. The HBM is further criticized for overlooking the fact that belief formation does not always precede behavioral change and that this causation relationship has the potential to be reversed (Haisch & Hornung, 2005; MSUCARES, 2001; Redding et al., 2000). Other theories such as the social support theory and gender power theories may fill in the void by explaining health behaviors rooted in social contexts, but in turn these theories often overlook influential cognitive factors such as beliefs and perceptions. For example, Durkheim's (1897/1951) study that links social support to health behavior is limited because its descriptive nature makes it fall short of an in-depth, qualitative-driven understanding of the meaning of sanctions pertaining to suicide across the two population groups under study. For example, the Catholic doctrine emphasizes eternal damnation for those who commit suicide, which is not the case for Protestants (Weber, 2002). The meaning of eternal damnation as a penalty may have been influential in determining suicide rates among the Catholic communities as opposed to the Protestant (Downes & Rock, 2003). Just as Durkheim's theory failed to exhaust all the possible predictors of suicide behavior in his study, the social support theory does not fully explain HAART adherence behavior.

In conclusion, none of the existing theories fully explains adherence behavior, especially in the social contexts seen in low-income countries such as sub-Saharan Africa. The most commonly used theory in this area is the HBM, which can be applied to HAART adherence in low-income nations. However, it is limited because it does not address behavior rooted in cultural or religious contexts, such as those related to gender power and poverty. The theory of gender power may explain condom use failure among females because of institutional economic, social, and political structures that render females powerless. Given their position in society, females often find themselves economically dependent on and subordinate to males such that they may fail to negotiate safe sex. Much of the work for females is in the domestic setting, and it is usually with meager or no compensation, which often renders females unable to comply with provider health care recommendations such as having a good diet or buying a condom. To a greater extent, combining the theory of gender power with the HBM may attempt to explain adherence behavior more fully in Uganda and other low-income nations. In any case, it remains a challenge for researchers to formulate a theory that integrates existing theories to exhaustively explain adherence behavior in low-income nations.

Chapter 3

Investigating HAART Adherence Behavior and Quality of Life

Purpose of the Study

The purpose of this study is to examine HAART adherence behavior, factors that influence adherence, and the impact of HAART on perceived quality of life for those under therapy. Information in this area is crucial because of the increasing effort on the part of the international community to scale up access to HAART in poor nations. The successful implementation of HAART requires adherence to medication regimens and to the HIV lifestyle recommendations such as condom use. Numerous studies conducted in this area in developed nations exist (e.g., Berg et al., 2007; Kalichman et al., 2001; Schonneson, Williams, Ross, Diamond, & Keel, 2007; Weidle et al., 2006). However, although the greatest impact of HIV/AIDS has been on developing nations, studies about adherence behavior as well as the physical and psychological effects of HAART on individuals in low-income countries are crucial but lacking (Badri, Wilson, & Wood, 2002; Ferradini et al., 2006; Mills et al., 2006; Schwartlander, Grubb, & Perriens, 2006). This study investigates just that. Some of the investigated areas in this study include: How are individuals on HAART adhering to treatment regimens? What factors influence highly active antiretroviral drug adherence behavior? What factors influence lifestyle recommendations adherence behavior? What is the impact of HAART on perceived physical and psychological health among individuals undergoing treatment? The following discusses the methodology for the study, including data collection and variable measurements.

Data and Data Collection

Data

Data utilized in this study consists of 70 client responses to a questionnaire collected in 2007. The questionnaire instrument measured adherence behavior and the impact of HAART on sexual behavior, as well as perceived physical and psychological health of Ugandan adults over age 18 who were currently enrolled in HAART.

Participants

Table 1 presents a summary of the main characteristics of the respondents. There were 70 participants in this study, all of whom were enrolled in HAART at the time data were collected. Of the respondents, 25 (37%) were soldiers and 45 (63%) were civilians. All participants were older than age 18. Based on this sample, the average age of participants was 37.6 with a standard deviation of 8.5. The youngest of the participants was 20 and the oldest 64 years of age; 92% of the respondents were younger than age 49. The average number of school years was 8.9 with a standard deviation of 3.9 and a range of 0 to 17 years of schooling. Forty-one percent of the respondents reported having only primary or no education. About 56% of the participants were female. Fifty-four percent of the respondents were married or cohabiting, 24% were widowed, and 22% never married or were separated. About 87% of the respondents were Christian, and 13% were Muslim. Of the participants, 86% indicated that they acquired HIV through heterosexual contact, 1% acquired it through blood transfusion, and 13% did not know how they contracted the virus. At the time of their enrollment in HAART, 60% of the respondents

TABLE 1. Characteristics of participants.

Measure	N	%	Mean/Median	SD
Age	70		37.6[a]	8.5
Years of Schooling	70		8.9[a]	3.9
Gender				
Male	31	44%		
Female	39	56%		
Marital				
Married/Cohabiting	29	41%		
Widowed	17	25%		
Never Married	24	34%		
Religion				
Christian	61	87%		
Muslim	9	13%		
Civil Status				
Civilians	44	63%		
Soldiers	26	37%		
CD4 Cell Count				
0–100	37	60%		
101–200	19	30%		
201+	6	10%		
Year Enrolled in HAART				
2000–2003	13	18%		
2004–2005	20	29%		
2006–2007	37	53%		
Transmission Mode				
Heterosexual Intercourse	60	86%		
Blood Transmission	1	1%		
Don't Know	9	13%		
Employment Status				
Employed	47	67%		
Unemployed	23	33%		
Monthly Family Income			$28[b] (U.S.)	
N	70			

Source. Data collected in Uganda, 2007.
[a] Mean.
[b] Median.

reported a CD4 cell count of below 100, 30% between 101 and 200, and 10% above 200. About 53% of the respondents began HAART between 2006 and 2007, 29% between 2004 and 2005, and 18% between 2000 and 2003. Thirty-three percent of the participants were unemployed; 67% were employed. Income ranged from $0 to $600 (U.S.) a month with a standard deviation of 7.6. The median income was $28 per month, with 59% of the respondents reporting earning less than $1 (U.S.) a day.

Recruitment of Participants

A convenience sampling technique was used to solicit participants because this technique appeared more feasible in terms of time and cost. Staff at the HAART-administering facilities played a major role in soliciting client participation by first informing those who met the inclusion criteria about the study and its purpose. Staff was requested to make an effort at creating a representative sample in terms of gender, age, and how long a respondent had been under therapy.

Instruments

I utilized questionnaires to collect data from the clients. These instruments were adapted from those developed by the DHHS. The questionnaire consisted of 119 closed-ended questions that measured and explored experiences with HAART, knowledge of highly active antiretroviral medications, HIV serostatus disclosure, medical outcomes, sexual behavior, alcohol use, and demographic characteristics. Questionnaires were first formulated in English and then developed in the Luganda language. English was used because it is the official language of Uganda. However, with the expectation that some participants may not understand English, a Luganda version of the questionnaire was prepared. Luganda was chosen because it is the most widely spoken native language in Uganda and is the native language in the area where the study was conducted.

Data Collection

All data were collected in a private setting to ensure confidentiality of participants, given the sensitive nature of the topic under study. In this setting, each participant was informed of the purpose as well as the potential risks and benefits of the study. Participants were also informed about the data collection procedure and that participation on their part was voluntary. To ensure maximum protection of confidentiality, verbal rather than written consent was obtained from clients.

A triangular approach was employed to collect data from clients on HAART. The triangular approach accommodated both quantitative and qualitative methods that would allow a deeper understanding of the social phenomena under study. A data collection strategy that combined both questionnaire and interview methods facilitated the triangular approach. Although it had been assumed that most of the data would be collected in English, 64 of the client questionnaires were completed in Luganda and only 6 were completed in English because many of the respondents could not understand, speak, or write English. Medication and lifestyle recommendations adherence behavior, their influential factors, and quality of life were measured.

Measuring Adherence Behavior

Following are nine indicators used to investigate how individuals on HAART adhered to treatment regimens: (a) skip dose, (b) on time, (c) condom use, (d) alcohol use, (e) sex partners, (f) good nutrition, (g) gender, (h) age, and (i) education. The coding discussion begins with original measures followed by the recoded measures. Skip dose and take on time were initially measured at ordinal levels using a 4-point Likert scale, with 1 for all the time, 2 for most of the time, 3 for sometimes, and 4 for never. Skip dose was dummy coded 1 for no, never skip a dose and 2 for yes, skips a dose. Similarly, on time was recoded 1 for no, does not always take medication on time, and 2 for yes, always takes it on time. Condom use was also originally measured at an ordinal level, with 1 for never use a condom, 2 for sometimes uses a condom, 3 for almost always uses a condom, and 4 for always uses a condom. Condom use was then recoded at a nominal level with 1 for no, does not use a condom regularly, and 2 for yes, always uses a condom. Alcohol was initially assessed by asking if respondent had an alcoholic beverage in the past

6 months; it was measured at a nominal level with 1 for no, never had an alcoholic drink, and 2 for yes, had an alcoholic drink. Alcohol was not recoded. Sex partners was initially measured at an interval ratio level by asking people to list the number of sex partners, but this was later recoded to a nominal level with 1 for have more than one sex partner and 2 for abstinence or one sex partner. Good nutrition was initially measured at an ordinal level with 1 for never has good nutrition, 2 for has good nutrition rarely, 3 for has good nutrition most of the time, and 4 for has good nutrition all the time. Good nutrition was then recoded 1 for no, does not always have good nutrition, and 2 for yes, always has good nutrition. Gender was coded 1 for female and 2 for male. Age of the respondent was initially measured at an interval ratio level but was later reduced to an ordinal level, with 1 for 20–29, 2 for 30–39, and 3 for 40–65. Similarly, education was originally measured at an interval ratio level but was later recoded at an ordinal level, with 1 for primary school or no education, 2 for senior or secondary school education, and 3 for higher school or college. One of the reasons for recoding measures from upper to lower levels of measurement was that the purpose of this question was to get a snapshot of two categories of people: those who completely comply with HAART regimens and those who do not. This knowledge would then be utilized as a foundation for the discussion of influential adherence factors in later research questions. In addition, it was necessary to get uniform measures that would allow fair comparisons across indicators. For example, skip dose was originally measured at an ordinal level using a 4-point Likert scale, with 1 for all the time, 2 for most of the time, 3 for sometimes, and 4 for never. However, alcohol was initially measured at a nominal level with 1 for no, never had an alcoholic drink in the past 6 months, and 2 for yes, had an alcoholic drink. Reducing skip dose to a nominal level and recoding it as 1 for no, never skips a dose, and 2 for yes, skips a dose, would allow comparison of skip dose and alcohol use because both indicators are measured at the nominal level. Another reason measures were reduced from higher to lower levels of measurement was to accommodate the use of cross tabulations that require analysis of variables with fewer categories.

Measuring Influential Antiretroviral Drug Adherence Behavior Factors

The nine indicators utilized to measure medication adherence behavior included (a) side effects, (b) alcohol, (c) embarrassment, (d) oversleeping, (e) forget to carry medication, (f) forget to take medication, (g) have no food, (h) social support, and (i) belief in effectiveness of highly active antiretroviral drugs. Asking if respondent skips taking medication because of side effects measured side effects. Alcohol was assessed by asking if respondent skips taking medication because of drinking alcohol. Asking if respondent skips taking medication because of embarrassment measured embarrassment. Oversleeping was assessed by asking if respondent skips taking medication because of sleeping through the dose. Forget to carry medication was measured by asking if respondent skips taking medication because of forgetting to carry it at all times. Asking if respondent skips taking medication because of forgetting measured forget to take medication. Have no food was measured by asking if respondent skips taking medication because of lack of food. All of the previous indicators were each initially measured at an ordinal level with 1 for skips all the time, 2 for skips most of the time, 3 for skips sometimes, and 4 for never skips. The same indicators were later recoded as 1 for no, never skips a dose, and 2 for yes, skips a dose. Asking if respondent has anyone to depend on for help taking medication assessed social support and was initially measured at a nominal level with 1 for no, has no social support, and 2 for yes, has social support. Social support was not recoded. Belief in effectiveness of highly active antiretroviral drugs in treating HIV was initially measured by responses to this statement: "I feel that if I keep taking my medication, my overall quality of life will definitely improve, probably improve, probably it may not improve, definitely it will not improve." This measure was recoded 1 for no, it will probably not improve or it will definitely not improve, and 2 for yes, it will probably improve or it will definitely improve. The major reason for recoding these indicators was to create uniform measures that would allow fair comparisons across indicators.

Measuring Influential Lifestyle Recommendations Adherence Factors

The four indicators employed to investigate factors that may influence lifestyle recommendations adherence behavior included (a) condom use, (b) number of sex partners, (c) alcohol use, and (d) good nutrition. Asking if respondent always uses a condom assesses condom use; it was originally measured at a nominal level with 1 for always uses a condom and 2 for does not always use a condom. Condom use was not recoded. Number of sex partners was initially measured at an interval ratio level by asking to state the number of sex partners a respondent has had since HAART initiation; this was recoded at a nominal level with 1 for abstinence or one sex partner and 2 for more than one sex partner. Alcohol use was originally measured by asking if respondent had an alcoholic drink in the last 6 months and it is measured at a nominal level with 1 for never had an alcoholic drink and 2 for yes, had an alcoholic drink. Alcohol was not recoded. Asking if respondent finds it hard to follow doctor's dietary recommendations assessed good nutrition; it was initially measured at an ordinal level, with 1 for never follows, 2 for follows rarely, 3 for follows most of the time, and 4 for follows all the time. Good nutrition was then recoded with 1 for no, does not always follow doctor's dietary recommendations, and 2 for yes, always follows dietary recommendations.

Measuring the Impact of HAART on Quality of Life

The three measures used to investigate perceived quality of life included (a) if respondent perceives physical health as much better, somewhat better, the same, or worse since HAART initiation; (b) if respondent perceives psychological health as much better, somewhat better, the same, or worse since HAART initiation; and (c) if respondent perceives overall quality of life as much better, somewhat better, the same, or worse since HAART initiation. All measures for the fourth research question were recoded as 1 for perceives health as somewhat better or much better and 2 for perceives health as the same as or worse than before HAART. It was necessary to recode these indicators to distinguish between two categories of people: those who perceived improvement in their quality of life since HAART initiation and those who perceived their health to be no different or worse than before HAART initiation.

Validity

All measurements were tested for validity to make sure that they measured exactly what they were intended to measure. Firstly, the questionnaire utilized was valid especially because it was adapted from the one used by a reputable organization—the DHHS—to measure HAART-adherence-related phenomenon in the United States. Some changes were made to make the instrument adaptable to the sub-Saharan social setting. Each item on the questionnaire was also examined to ensure face validity. Additionally, construct validity was used to note the extent to which each measure performed according to the theoretical expectations of adherence behavior. For example, on the basis of prior literature, it is expected that females are less likely to use condoms as compared to males. In that regard, construct validity of gender as a measure of adherence was assessed to see if a positive relationship between gender and adherence behavior emerged.

Data Analysis

The instrument used to collect data from clients was composed of both open- and closed-ended questions that facilitate quantitative and qualitative analysis. Data from all open-ended questions to a questionnaire were transcribed, processed, and entered into the computer. Processing of clients' open-ended responses included language translation from Luganda to English, response clarification, and grammatical error cleaning while keeping as much of the original information as possible. Similarly, questionnaire responses to the closed-ended questions were entered into a computer statistical software package, after which the quantitative data was cleaned, coded, and stored for accurate analysis.

Quantitative Data Analysis

Because the sample size was small ($N = 70$ clients), elementary quantitative data analysis was utilized. Descriptive statistics were used to analyze distribution patterns and the general characteristics of data. Cross tabulations were used in order to get some understanding of the structure of adherence behavior, especially with reference to gender, education, and age. Phi and Cranmer's V were employed to analyze the significance, strength, and direction of associations between adherence measures and gender, education, and age. The reason for choosing phi and Cranmer's V was that most of the measures under analysis were measured at nominal levels. The analysis was limited to adherence behavior and gender, education, and age because cross-tabulation results revealed no differences between adherence behavior and other demographic characteristics such as religion. Scholars agree that many of the demographic factors are not good predictors of adherence behavior (Williams & Friedland, 1997).

Qualitative Data Analysis

Qualitative data analysis techniques were also employed to decode major themes pertaining to influential HAART adherence factors and the impact of HAART on health. Concepts and themes in the data set were coded while noting theoretical revelations as they unfolded. An inductive approach was used in the qualitative analysis, beginning with specific observations and continuing into the discovery of patterns.

Limitations of the Study

One of the limitations of this study was the use of the convenience sampling technique. As a result, the findings cannot be generalized beyond the population group or geographical area investigated in this study. Participants in this study were also affiliated with the centers from where the data were collected. Participant and service provider relationship issues may have had an effect on the validity of the information. Because of time and financial constraints, the sample size in this study is small ($N = 70$). A small sample size does not favor the utilization of more advanced statistical techniques. In addition, some of the measures pertain to sensitive personal issues, such as sexual behavior. This may also raise reliability and validity concerns because of fear of the negative social stigma associated with certain sexual behaviors, such as engagement in sex with multiple partners while HIV positive.

Another limitation is that the majority of the interviews were conducted in Luganda, and they were translated in English for analysis. The translation process has a potential of losing some information. However, I personally collected all the data. As a native born in Uganda who has lived in the social, economic, and cultural context of the participants, I tried as much as possible to maintain the original meaning of the responses, not only in reference to language but in conjunction with the perceived nonverbal communication of the respondents. It is also important to note that the data is limited to a cross-sectional design such that changes in reference to the impact of HAART, adherence, medical outcomes, and behavioral changes over time cannot be investigated. Despite the limitations, to a great extent, findings in this study present an accurate current picture of HAART adherence behavior and quality of life for the population under study. As revealed further on, the benefits from findings in this study significantly outweigh its limitations.

Chapter 4

The Impact of HAART Adherence on Quality of Life

The previous chapter discussed the methodology of the study and presented measurements for HAART adherence and quality of life for those under therapy in Uganda. This chapter presents quantitative and qualitative analytical findings of data from 70 participants that portray distribution patterns of the four investigated areas—beginning with HAART adherence behavior, followed by factors that influence medication adherence behavior and factors that influence lifestyle recommendations adherence behavior, and ending with the impact of HAART on perceived quality of life.

HAART Adherence Behavior

The first area of investigation was how individuals on HAART in Uganda are adhering to medication regimens as well as to health provider lifestyle recommendations. It is important to obtain a better understanding of HAART adherence behavior among those undergoing therapy in low-income nations such as Uganda because such information may lead to the formulation of strategies necessary to enhance compliance with HAART and thus the effective implementation of HAART to improve the quality of life for those under therapy. Several questions asked to investigate adherence behavior among Ugandan adults included the following: Are individuals on HAART taking medication as prescribed in terms of dosing and timing? Are people on HAART adhering to lifestyle recommendations such as safe sex, abstinence from alcohol, and good nutrition? Who is more or less likely to adhere to medication regimens? Who is more or less likely to adhere to lifestyle recommendations? As detailed in chapter 3, indicators employed to measure HAART adherence included skip dose, on time, condom use, alcohol use, sex partners, good nutrition, gender, age, and education. However, before proceeding, it is necessary to define some of the terms used to investigate adherence behavior, such as "skipping taking a dose" and "taking medication on time." Skipping taking medication means that the patient completely misses taking a given dose of medication. For instance, if medication is scheduled to be taken twice daily, the patient may skip a dose and take medication only once a day instead of twice or even skip taking both doses. In contrast, failure to take medication on time means that the patient does not skip taking a dose of medication but takes it a few hours before or after the scheduled time.

Adherence behavior is presented by first giving the overall pattern for all participants, followed by a comparison of findings across gender, age, and education level of the respondents. As detailed later, findings reveal that females are more likely to skip taking medication and less likely to use a condom as compared to males. Males instead are less likely to take medication on time, more likely to have more than one sex partner, and more likely to use alcohol as compared to females. Younger individuals are more likely to skip taking medication and to drink alcohol than their older counterparts. Less educated individuals are more likely to skip taking medication and not using a condom as compared to the more educated. The more educated are more likely not to take medication on time, to have sex with multiple partners, and to drink alcohol as compared to the less educated.

Noteworthy is the fact that although some of the findings are insignificant, I have included them in the discussion because the relationships portrayed are generally consistent with findings in the literature. Additionally, despite the fact that religion has the potential to reveal interesting adherence behavioral patterns, specifically in the analysis of Muslims versus Christians, it is not included in this study because few participants ($n = 9$) indicate they are Muslim as compared to those who indicate they belong to the Christian faith ($n = 60$). That is, if religion is included as a predictor for adherence, the unequal representation of both groups could lead to biased results.

As shown in table 2, a general view of findings reveals that respondents were almost equally divided between those who always took medication on time (51%) and those who did not always take medication on time (49%). In addition, 41% of the participants indicated that they sometimes skipped taking medication, whereas 59% reported that they never skipped taking medication. These results may be of concern to public health as discussed before because adherence failure creates the danger of the formation of drug-resistant HIV. Furthermore, of all lifestyle recommendations, respondents were least likely to report having good nutrition, as most (83%) reported failure to follow doctor's orders of ensuring good nutrition. Only 17% of the respondents reported that they always had good nutrition. Failure to have good nutrition may be partially attributed to financial need. That is, as portrayed in the descriptive statistical results of study participants presented in chapter 3, although 67% of the respondents stated that they were employed, the median income of participants was only $28 (U.S.) a month, with about 60% of the respondents reporting earnings of less than $1 a day. Table 2 also reveals that adherence behavior with regard to practicing safe sex and abstaining from alcohol was better than that of medication regimens: a large majority (84%) of respondents reported either having sex with only one partner or abstaining from sex, and more than half (60%) reported using condoms regularly. A large number of participants (62%) also reported abstinence from alcohol. Following the general overview of findings for all participants are analytical findings of adherence behavior across demographic characteristics.

TABLE 2. Measures of adherence behavior.

Item	*N*	%
Medications Adherence Behavior		
Skips Taking Medication		
Sometimes or Always Skips	28	40.6
Never Skips	41	59.4
Total	69	100.0
Takes Medication on Time		
Sometimes or Never	34	48.6
Always	36	51.4
Total	70	100.0
Lifestyle Adherence Behavior		
Uses Condoms		
Does Not Always Use	19	40.4
Always Uses	28	59.6
Total	47	100.0
Abstains or Has One Sex Partner		
Does Not Abstain/Has More Than One Partner	11	15.7
Abstains or Has One Partner	59	84.3
Total	70	100.0
Abstains From Alcohol		
Had at Least One Drink	26	37.7
Abstains	43	62.3
Total	69	100.0
Has Good Nutrition		
Not Always	58	82.9
Always	12	17.1
Total	70	100.0

Source. Data collected in Uganda, 2007.

Adherence Behavior Across Sex

Results pertaining to adherence behavior by sex are shown in table 3, and they reveal that overall, males were less likely to comply with health providers' medication regimens than females. For example, about 58% of the males indicated that they did not take medication on time as compared to 41% of the females. This could partially be attributed to the fact that males are usually more involved in the labor force than females, who usually take on domestic roles or are unemployed. That is, there is potential for some males to forget taking medication on time when busy at work. Males were also less likely to comply with abstinence from sex and alcohol or to have one sex partner. For instance, males (52%) were twice as likely as females (26%) to report having used alcohol in the last 6 months. More males (19%) also reported having multiple sex partners than females (13%). One of the major reasons why more men may engage in sex with multiple partners as compared to females may be the cultural context from which the study was conducted, a culture that encourages polygamy for procreation purposes. However, more females (47%) reported skipping taking medication as compared to males (32%). Skipping taking medication on the part of females may be partially attributed to economic constraints. That is, females are usually either engaged in domestic roles or unemployed or if in the labor force generally underpaid such that although medication is free, they may not be able to afford food required to take medication if recommended on a full stomach. In the same vein, females may also fail to get transportation to clinics for refills, which may lead to skipping taking medication between prescription refills.

Furthermore, females (42%) were also more likely to report failure to use a condom regularly as compared to males (39%). This could be attributed to gender imbalances embedded in the cultural context in which the study was conducted, a culture that renders females powerless to make safe sex decisions such as using a condom. In contrast, gender differences in following the doctor's orders to have good nutrition were negligible. Moreover, except for alcohol and gender, the associations between gender and failure to use a condom as discussed earlier

Table 3. Adherence behavior by sex.

Item	Gender				
	Male		*Female*		
	N	*%*	*N*	*%*	*Phi*
Medication Adherence Behavior					
Skips Taking Medication					.153
Sometimes or Always	10	32.3	18	47.4	
Never Skips	21	67.7	20	52.6	
Total	31	100.0	38	100.0	
Takes Medication on Time					–.169
Sometimes or Never	18	58.1	16	41.0	
Always	13	41.9	23	59.0	
Total	31	100.0	39	100.0	
Lifestyle Adherence Behavior					
Uses Condoms					.028
Does Not Always Use	11	39.3	8	42.1	
Always Uses	17	60.7	11	57.9	
Total	28	100.0	19	100.0	
Abstains or Has One Sex Partner					–.089
Does Not Abstain/Has More Than One Partner	6	19.4	5	12.8	
Abstains or Has One Partner	25	80.6	34	87.2	
Total	31	100.0	39	100.0	
Abstains From Alcohol					–.260*
Had at Least One Drink	16	51.6	10	26.3	
Abstains	15	48.4	28	73.7	
Total	31	100.0	38	100.0	
Has Good Nutrition					–.024
Not Always	26	83.9	32	82.1	
Always	5	16.1	7	17.9	
Total	31	100.0	39	100.0	

Source. Data collected in Uganda, 2007.
* = $p < .05$.

are weak and insignificant at the 0.05 level, even though other scholars reveal somewhat similar results.

Adherence Behavior by Age

Investigation of adherence behavior by age reveals that HAART adherence failure is more common among younger individuals than their older counterparts. For example, results in table 4 show that the largest percentage of those who reported skipping taking a dose of medication was for individuals between ages 20 and 29 (50%), followed by respondents between ages 30 and 39 (47%). One thing that may explain this pattern could be that older people possess better medication-taking experiences as compared to the young. Table 4 also clearly indicates that the youngest age group (ages 20 to 29) was far more likely to fail to adhere to abstinence from alcohol (73%) than those over age 40 (only 33% reported failure to adhere by drinking alcohol). Similarly, younger people were also more likely to fail to comply with dietary regimens (92% report failure to comply) than older respondents, suggesting perhaps a lack of resources to purchase food. Moreover, more individuals ages 30 to 39 (46%) and those over age 40 (40%) reported failure to use condoms on a regular basis as compared to those under 30 years of age (25%). One of the reasons failure to use condoms was higher among those over age 30 than those under age 30 may be partly that those over age 30 are more likely to be married than those younger. The institution of marriage is often followed by a desire to procreate. Unfortunately for HIV-positive individuals, condoms have the potential to prevent pregnancy. Another concern for those over age 30 interested in procreation could be that fertility may decline with age, which has potential to create panic for those who feel they may not be able to bear children once they reach a certain age. Furthermore, individuals over age 40 (52%) were also less likely to take medication on time as compared to those ages 20 to 29 (42%). In investigating adherence behavior across age, the association between alcohol use and age group is significant and moderately strong (phi = 0.318, $p < .05$). Other associations are not significant but are consistent with those found in the literature.

Table 4. Adherence behavior by age.

Item	Age						
	20–29		30–39		40–65		
	N	%	*N*	%	*N*	%	*Phi*
Medication Adherence Behavior							
Skips Taking Medication							.180
Sometimes or Always	6	50.0	14	46.7	8	29.6	
Never Skips	6	50.0	16	53.3	19	70.4	
Total	12	100.0	30	100.0	27	100.0	
Takes Medication on Time							.070
Sometimes or Never	5	41.7	15	48.4	14	51.9	
Always	7	58.3	16	51.6	13	48.1	
Total	12	100.0	31	100.0	27	100.0	
Lifestyle Adherence Behavior							
Uses Condoms							.152
Does Not Always	2	25.0	11	45.8	6	40.0	
Always Uses	6	75.0	13	54.2	9	60.0	
Total	8	100.9	24	100.0	15	100.0	

Abstains or Has One Sex Partner							.020
Does Not Abstain/Has More Than One Partner	2	16.7	5	16.1	4	14.8	
Abstains or Has One Partner	10	83.3	26	83.9	23	85.2	
Total	12	100.0	31	100.0	27	100.0	
Abstains From Alcohol							.318*
Had at Least One Drink in Last 6 Months	8	72.7	9	29.0	9	33.3	
Abstains	3	27.3	22	71.0	18	66.7	
Total	11	100.0	31	100.0	27	100.0	
Has Good Nutrition							–.142
Not Always	11	91.7	24	77.4	23	85.2	
Always	1	8.3	7	22.6	4	14.8	
Total	12	100.0	31	100.0	27	100.0	

Source. Data collected in Uganda, 2007.
* = $p < .05$.

Adherence Behavior by Education Level

The investigation of adherence behavior by education level is presented in table 5. Based on the findings, less educated individuals were more likely to skip taking medication and more likely to report failure to use condoms regularly as compared to those who are more educated. For example, nearly half (48%) of those with no education or only primary school education reported skipping a dose of medication, as compared to only 13% of those with higher schooling or college. This trend is also true of condom use (table 5), whereby individuals with no or primary school education were almost five times as likely (68%) as those with college education (14%) to report failure to use a condom regularly. The relationship between education level and condom use is moderately strong and significant (phi = .474, $p < .05$). In contrast, the percentage of more educated people who reported using alcohol (38%) is higher than those of individuals with primary education (28%), probably for economic reasons. That is, the more educated are more likely to possess the means to obtain alcohol and, if males, to have sex with several partners as compared to the less educated. Generally males are expected to have more education than females, and it may be true that the more education one achieves, the better the occupation and the higher the income. In social contexts where many of the poor are females, some women may engage in sex for financial assistance, often received from males. Nevertheless, pertaining to adherence behavior across education, except for condom use and education level, other associations are weak and insignificant.

In summary, the percentage of respondents who reported always taking medication on time (51%) and those who reported failure to always take medication on time (49%) is almost equal. About 60% of the respondents reported that sometimes they skip taking a dose. Furthermore, a comparison of adherence behavior across gender, age, and education reveals that males are less likely to comply with the health provider's treatment regimens as opposed to females. On the one hand, males were more likely to have multiple sex partners, to drink alcohol for cultural reasons, and not to take medication on time. Females, on the other hand, were less likely to use condoms regularly because they lack power to negotiate safe

TABLE 5. Adherence behavior by education level.

Item	Education Level: None/ Primary School N	%	Senior School N	%	College/ University N	%	Phi
Medications Adherence Behavior							
Skips Taking Medication							.220
Sometimes or Always	14	48.3	13	40.6	1	12.5	
Never Skips	15	51.7	19	59.4	7	87.5	
Total	29	100.0	32	100.0	8	100.0	
Takes Medication on Time							.138
Sometimes or Never	12	41.4	17	51.5	5	62.5	
Always	17	58.6	16	48.5	3	37.5	
Total	29	100.0	33	100.0	8	100.0	
Lifestyle Adherence Behavior							
Uses Condoms							.474*
Does Not Always Use	13	68.4	5	23.8	1	14.3	
Always Uses	6	31.6	16	76.2	6	85.7	
Total	19	100.0	21	100.0	7	100.0	
Abstains or Has One Sex Partner							.144
Does Not Abstain/Has More Than One Partner	3	10.3	7	21.2	1	12.5	
Abstains or Has One Partner	26	89.7	26	78.8	7	87.5	
Total	29	100.0	33	100.0	8	100.0	
Abstains from Alcohol							.187
Had at Least One Drink in Last 6 Months	8	27.6	15	46.9	3	37.5	
Abstains	21	72.4	17	53.1	5	62.5	
Total	29	100.0	32	100.0	8	100.0	
Has Good Nutrition							.171
Not Always	24	82.8	26	78.8	8	100.0	
Always	5	17.2	7	21.2	0	0.00	
Total	29	100.0	33	100.0	8	100.0	

Source. Data collected in Uganda, 2007.
* = $p < .05$.

sex. Older people used condoms less than younger individuals probably because they were more likely to engage in monogamous relationships. However, overall younger people were less likely to adhere to medication regimes and lifestyle recommendations as compared to their older counterparts. Additionally, less educated individuals reported sometimes skipping taking medication and not using a condom regularly more than people with higher education, possibly because they do not fully understand the public health implications of HAART adherence failure. In contrast, more educated people report using alcohol and having sex with multiple partners more than those with primary or no education, probably because of economic reasons.

Factors That Influence Antiretroviral Drug Adherence Behavior

Adherence behavioral patterns across demographic characteristics have been presented in the previous sections, and they reveal that some individuals are failing to adhere to health providers' recommendations. The second investigated area pertains to what influences anti-HIV drug adherence behavior among Ugandan adults on HAART. As stated before, medication adherence for those under HAART is important because failure to comply with prescription regimens may lead to the formation of drug-resistant HIV that cannot be controlled by existing anti-HIV medication (Machtinger & Bangsberg, 2008; Wensing & Boucher, 2003). Crucial to investigate is why some individuals on HAART fail to adhere to medication regimens and what makes others comply. Findings from the study may help health providers assist those undergoing therapy, specifically in low-income nations, adapt better medication adherence practices. In addition, findings may assist in the efficient distribution of resources geared toward enhancement of HAART effectiveness in developing countries. Data analyzed in this area yielded the following results. The analyzed results are based on nine measures predicting influential medication adherence factors as presented in chapter 3. These predictors include side effects, alcohol, embarrassment, oversleeping, forgetting to carry medication, forgetting to take medication, having no food, social support, and belief in effectiveness of medication.

Based on findings revealed in table 6, lack of food was the major obstacle for skipping taking medication as reported by 59% of the respondents, followed by forgetting to carry medication while traveling (33%). Although studies conducted in developed countries reveal that

TABLE 6. Factors influencing adherence behavior.

Item	*N*	%
Medication-Related Factors		
Side Effects		
Sometimes or Always Skip Due to Side Effects	1	1.8
Never Skip Due to Side Effects	55	98.2
Total	56	100.0
Alcohol Use		
Sometimes or Always Skip Due to Alcohol Use	4	6.3
Never Skip Due to Alcohol Use	60	93.8
Total	64	100.0
Embarrassment		
Sometimes or Always Skip Due to Embarrassment	10	15.6
Never Skip Due to Embarrassment	54	84.4
Total	64	100.0
Oversleeping		
Sometimes Skip Due to Oversleeping	11	17.2
Never Skip Due to Oversleeping	53	82.8
Total	64	100.0
Forget to Carry Medication		
Sometimes or Always Skip Due to Forgetting to Carry	13	18.6
Never Skip Due to Forgetting to Carry	57	81.4
Total	70	100.0

(*continued on the next page*)

TABLE 6. *(continued)*

Item	*N*	%
Forget to Take Medication		
Sometimes or Always Skip Due to Forgetting	22	33.3
Never Skip Due to Forgetting	44	66.7
Total	66	100.0
Have No Food		
Sometimes or Always Skip Due to No Food	41	58.6
Never Skip Due to No Food	29	41.4
Total	70	100.0
Other Influential Factors		
Has Social Support		
No Social Support	13	18.6
Has Social Support	57	81.4
Total	70	100.0
Believes in Effectiveness of Medication		
Probably or Definitely Will Help	69	98.6
Probably or Definitely Will Not Help	1	1.4
Total	70	100.0

Source. Data collected in Uganda, 2007.

side effects influence medication adherence failure, findings in this study show that side effects had the least influence on skipping taking medication, with only 2% of the participants reporting that they sometimes skipped taking medication because of side effects (Ammassari et al., 2001; Safren et al., 2005). An overwhelming majority (98%) indicated that they take medication regardless of side effects. Likewise, 94% of the participants reported that alcohol use does not make them skip taking medication. A large percentage of respondents also indicated that embarrassment (84%), sleeping through the dose (83%), and not carrying medication (81%) do not make them skip taking medication, which shows that these issues have minimal impact on medication adherence behavior among those under HAART in Uganda. Medication representation may explain the high percentages of adherence as indicated here because almost all participants (99%) reported that they believed their overall quality of life would improve if they kept taking highly active antiretroviral drugs. As revealed in chapter 2, belief in the effectiveness of medication or medication representation is highlighted in literature as influential in medication adherence behavior (Garcia & Cote, 2003). The presence of social support may also partially explain the high percentages of those who claim to adhere to medication regimens. Research reveals that lack of social support may enhance adherence failure (Munro et al., 2007). The results in this study show that more than three quarters of the respondents (81%) had someone they depended on to (help them) take medication. In addition to quantitative responses, participants were also given an opportunity to explain why they fail to adhere to medication regimens. Following is the qualitative analysis of their responses.

Skipping or Not Skipping Taking Medication

When participants were asked specifically to explain why they skip taking medication, lack of food, fear of mixing alcohol with medication, and doctor communication emerged as the major themes. Previous experiences with opportunistic diseases, illness and medication representation, and confidence and trust in the doctor also surfaced as major reasons for adherence to medication regimens.

Why Individuals Skip Taking Medication

A dominant theme that emerged when respondents were asked to explain why they sometimes skip taking medication was lack of food. Most of those who reported skipping taking medication because of lack of food often expressed the desire to take medication but at the same time feelings of helplessness to take it regularly because they did not have the economic means to buy food. For instance, these feelings are detected in a 28-year-old female participant's statement when she claimed,

> I do not want to miss taking medication. However, the doctor tells me to take it on a full stomach, yet at times I do not have money to buy food. When I have no food to eat that is when I skip taking medication. Otherwise merely swallowing the tablet is not an issue because I can easily and willingly do that.

A 30-year-old female participant also relayed feelings of helplessness to adhere to the health providers' dietary recommendations as she indicated, "I would rather the doctor does not put the food condition on taking medicine because if you have no food, then you may skip taking your medicine."

Males also reported skipping taking medication because of lack of food. For example, a 36-year-old male respondent claimed, "I sometimes miss taking medicine because I have no food to eat before I take it. In Africa we have a general problem of following the doctors' orders to take medication with food because of low income."

Fear of mixing alcohol with highly active antiretroviral drugs was another theme that surfaced as a reason for skipping medication. Some of the participants revealed that they skipped taking medication intentionally when they were under the influence of alcohol because of HAART education. For example, a 45-year-old respondent justified his medication taking behavior by saying,

> When I take alcohol, I do not swallow medication because the health providers informed me it is dangerous to mix alcohol with medication as it may turn medicine into poison. They also told me that medicine does not work well if it finds alcohol in the system and I understood that. Therefore, when I drink alcohol, I find it justified skipping a dose as I reason within myself that, if I take the medication, I will be wasting it. Skipping that dose makes me feel I have done the right thing.

Another male respondent also conveyed this theme in a more explicit way when he said,

> When I drink, I intentionally skip taking mediation because the doctor told me that I can't mix spirits with medical drugs. In that case when I feel a craving for an alcoholic drink, I have to make a choice if it is the drink or medication. If I decide to cheat by taking alcohol, then I take the drink and not the medicine.

Other participants indicated that skipping taking medication after drinking alcohol is not intentional, but they forget to take medication while under the influence of alcohol. For example, as a 31-year-old male soldier confessed, "When my friends join me, I'm forced to drink alcohol with them. The problem is that drinking often makes me forget taking medication."

Why Individuals Do Not Skip Taking Medication

Of the 59% who indicated they never skip taking a dose, previous experiences with opportunistic diseases, illness and medication representation, and trust in the doctor emerged as major influences for not skipping taking medication. Illness representation in this discussion refers to individual beliefs about HIV and medication representation to beliefs about the effect of medicine on HIV. The influence of illness and medication representation on not skipping taking medication may be detected in a 25-year-old female respondent's statement:

> I do not find any difficulty following the doctor's orders to take medication in a given dose at the exact time because, based on my experiences with opportunistic illnesses, if someone tells me that this medication will soothe the pain, I swallow it immediately without question. This is because I cannot explain to you the pain I experienced from some of the opportunistic illnesses before I started HAART…I do exactly as the doctor tells me to do.

The influence of medication representation on adherence is also detected in a 35-year-old female participant's affirmation:

> I have no problem following the doctor's orders because, in comparison to the situation I was in before I began HAART, I have hope that my health will continue improving. I know this because

> I feel energetic and I am no longer sickly as I used to be before I began HAART.

Males also portrayed experiences with opportunistic illness as well as illness and medication representation to be influential in not skipping taking medication. For example, a 45-year-old male respondent asserted,

> I do not skip taking medication because I see a change in my life. For seven years before I started HAART, I was often down with various illnesses, feeling extremely ill and completely under the control of AIDS. However, when I began HAART I decided to comply with the doctor's advice. I was told to eat, drink, and use medications as prescribed and I complied. My health improved month after month. Currently I feel that my health is good.

Confidence and trust in the doctor was another theme that surfaced in explaining why individuals do not skip taking medication. The influence of health providers on adherence is depicted in a 45-year-old male respondent's statement:

> I take medication as prescribed because my doctor convinced me to do so. For example, he asked me to tell him my age and I told him I am forty-three years of age. He then informed me that if I keep taking this medication as prescribed, I will be able to add thirty more years to my life's span and I was extremely happy. For that reason alone I try not to skip a dose.

A 32-year-old female also stressed,

> I follow the doctor's orders because I believe whatever he says is true. He told me to take the medication all the time and when I did, I got better. He told me not to drink alcohol and I stopped. He told me to use a condom and I do because I realize there is a change in my life.

Taking or Failure to Take Medication on Time

Additionally, table 2 shows that about half (49%) of the respondents indicated they sometimes did not take medication on time, whereas the other half (51%) revealed they always took it on time. Failing to take medication on time minimizes HAART's effectiveness in treating HIV because, as discussed in chapter 2, it lowers the required drug concentration level in the blood system, giving HIV the chance to mutate and multiply (Descamps et al., 2000). In an attempt to further understand what influences individual medication-taking behavior, respondents were asked to explain in depth why they did or did not take medication on time. This led to the emergence of various themes, such as stigma, being busy, and traveling. In contrast, choosing a convenient time, cues to action, and disclosure emerged as influential factors in taking medication on time. These emergent themes are discussed in the following paragraphs.

Why Individuals Fail to Take Medication on Time

Fear of stigma was reported as one of the main reasons why individuals did not take medication on time, with respondents often expressing fear of ridicule. Because of the HIV stigma, individuals are afraid to disclose to others their HIV status, which they want to keep confidential, especially from the public. For example, a 28-year-old female participant revealed,

> Sometimes I fail to take medication at the appointed time because I cannot find a way to get away from other people to take it, especially at work. In such cases, I just have to wait for that time when I can be alone to take it...I conceal taking my medication, and in so doing fail to take it at the appointed time.

Another theme highlighted by numerous respondents as an obstacle to taking medication on time was being busy, which may lead to forgetfulness to take medicine. A 34-year-old female respondent who expounded on this theme stated, "I sometimes fail to take medication on time. For example, I may be attending a business meeting and time may elapse unnoticed such that I may forget it is time to take medication."

As another female respondent put it, "I forget to take medication on time when I get so busy at work. However, I take it as soon as I remember."

Traveling away from home without taking medication along also surfaced as an influential factor in failure to take medication on time. For instance, a female respondent stated,

> I sometimes fail to take medication on time if I travel. For example, I may go to the village to visit family or for a funeral and by the time I get back in town, the time to take my evening dose has elapsed.

Why Individuals Take Medication on Time

Of the 51% who indicated they always take medication on time, choosing a convenient time and cues to action, as well as disclosure, emerged as influential factors for the timely intake of medication. For example, a 44-year-male respondent who was given a choice to decide a time to take medication confidently stated,

> I always take my medication on time because the doctor allowed me to choose a convenient time to take it and I chose nine o'clock in morning and evening. At nine o'clock in the morning, I have taken morning tea such that the next thing I do is to take medication. At nine o'clock in the evening I am home and before I go to bed, I take the medication. Therefore, I see no reason for not taking my medication on time.

Likewise, a 24-year-old female participant was given a choice to decide a time to take the medication and chose a convenient time with a cue to action; she stated,

> I have no difficulty taking medication on time because the doctor told me to choose the most convenient time to take it and I chose nine o'clock in the morning and evening. Nine o'clock is time for the national news broadcast such that, whenever I hear the news on radio regardless of what I am doing, I know it is time to take my medication such that I just go and take it.

Physical pain as a cue to take medication on time was also mentioned as a factor influencing adherence to medication regimens. As a 26-year-old female indicated,

> When I take long without taking medication, I feel as if my stomach is beginning to hurt. However, as soon as I try to take the medication like this, the pain in my stomach disappears immediately. That means I have to take medication on time. If I go five minutes past that time my stomach begins to unravel and to hurt. However, as soon as I take the medication like this, the rumbling stops immediately.

Disclosure was another theme. Individuals who disclosed their serostatus to others, or who felt that other people knew they were HIV positive, indicated that they had nothing to hide by concealing taking medication, which meant that they were able to always take medication on time and anywhere. The relation between disclosure and always taking medication on time was revealed in this statement from one of the female participants:

> I have no problem at all taking medication on time or before other people because most of my relatives and friends know that I have AIDS. I was forced to tell them because I developed *kisipi* [slang for herpes zoster], which made it obvious to all who saw me that I have AIDS. For that reason, I have nothing to hide by concealing medication intake because people already know I have AIDS.

Side Effects and Skipping Taking Medication

Research also reveals that adherence failure is more likely for those who perceive medication to cause undesirable side effects (Berg et al., 2007; Hardon et al., 2007). Gao et al.'s (2000) study reported that side effects from medications are the greatest perceived obstacle to taking medication regularly. However, as revealed in table 6, despite the fact that some of the side effects caused by highly active antiretroviral drugs may be severe, when respondents in this study were asked specifically if side effects sometimes made them skip taking medication, almost all participants (98%) said side effects did not make them skip taking medication. Only 2% indicated side effects sometimes make them skip taking medication. Asked to support their responses, almost all participants who indicated side effects to be an obstacle in taking medication indicated that health provider communication and previous experiences with opportunistic infections were the factors that most influenced their medication-taking behavior. For instance, a 30-year-old female participant who had been on HAART for less than 3 months and who was experiencing numerous side effects concurrently explained,

> Since I started taking this medication, I experience side effects often in the form of headaches, dizziness…and nightmares. However, I do not skip taking my medication because I was warned by the doctor that these health conditions are expected, and that they usually disappear within three to six months.

Another female participant who portrayed the influence of doctor communication on medication adherence regardless of side effects manifestations also claimed,

> Taking highly active antiretroviral drugs makes me nauseated. However, nausea does not stop me from taking medication because the doctor told me that it is normal to experience side effects for those under HAART. Sometimes I may throw up after taking the medication. However, when that happens I don't re-take it because the doctor did not inform me how medicine reacts after it has been in the body for thirty minutes.

Male respondents were also adamant about taking medication regardless of side effects, which is attributed to doctor communication as well. For instance, as a 30-year-old male respondent emphasized,

> There is no time that I get sick and fail to take medication. Whatever illness hits, I swallow the medication because the doctor insisted that it is important I keep taking it regardless of side effects because they are temporary, and that they only last for a few months.

Embarrassment and Skipping Taking Medication

According to the literature, embarrassment or shame may be an obstacle to medication adherence whereby individuals may skip or fail to take medication on time if the timing for taking it finds them in the company of other people (Wurth & Perlow, 2005). When asked specifically if respondents sometimes skip taking medication because of embarrassment, the majority (84%) of the respondents reported they never skip, indicating that the influence of embarrassment on taking medication is minimal. Some participants stated that disclosure had a big influence on whether they sometimes skipped taking medication or not while others are watching. Participants who reported skipping taking medication as a result of embarrassment expressed concerns for HIV/AIDS stigma and social setting; whereas value for life, perception that HIV can infect anyone, and belief that spectators can't tell the type of medication one is taking surfaced as influential factors for those who complied with medication regimens in spite of being watched by others. Following is an elaborated account of adherence behavior and embarrassment responses.

Skipping Taking Medication Due to Embarrassment

One of the reasons indicated for skipping taking medication because of embarrassment was HIV/AIDS stigma. This can be detected in some participants' responses, as quoted next. For example, a 27-year-old female respondent who reported sometimes skipping medication because of embarrassment and who expressed concerns for stigma explained,

> I find it difficult to take medication when others are watching and if possible I usually excuse myself and go into the back where no one can see me because AIDS is stigmatized. If I can't excuse myself, I may miss a dose or take it late. Another way that I hide my medication use, I may decide to swallow it on the way from work before I get home in order to avoid others from seeing me take it. However, this is usually before the appointed time for taking that particular dose.

Male respondents also expressed concern with stigma, shame, and disclosure. As a 36-year-old male respondent asserted,

> I keep my medication in the bedroom such that only my wife and I know about it. You cannot put that medication in the office and take it when other people are watching because you can't go

> reporting yourself by spreading the word to everyone that I am sick, I am sick, I have AIDS. It is like putting your business on the table for everyone to see.

Numerous participants also implicated social setting as having an influence on whether they sometimes skipped taking medication. Some individuals revealed that they were embarrassed or ashamed to take medication in certain environments. This is seen in a statement made by a 49-year-old male respondent:

> I wouldn't take medication when other people are looking like at work because people do not understand, which sometimes makes me skip taking it. However, I can take it openly at this clinic [HAART-providing clinic] without a problem because I know that people here share the same problem as I do.

Other participants reported that among those to whom they had not disclosed, they did not always take medication regularly. For instance, as reported by a 25-year-old female respondent,

> When the people I am with do not know that I am HIV positive, I have difficulty taking antiretroviral medication, and I may fail to take it. I can't show my medication to everyone. For example, one person may notice you are swallowing medication. The next thing you may hear is that, "that person is at the end of the road [*aweddeyo*]." The funny thing is that, those that gossip may even fail to realize the possibility that they could die from any other health condition before I do.

A 27-year-old female participant also identified concerns for disclosure and stigma by stating,

> At times I may skip taking medication because I am embarrassed to take it before other people. I don't care for those I have disclosed to, but there are other people for example at work that I don't want to notice I am taking highly active antiretroviral drugs... If people like that find out you have AIDS, they start back-biting you. Because of that, I often use wisdom to make sure others do

> not see me taking antiretroviral medication, but in so doing I may take it late.

Taking Medication Regardless of Embarrassment

Disclosure was also used positively in explaining why individuals comply with medication regimens. Other influential factors included prioritizing value for life before embarrassment, perception of AIDS as affecting everyone, and belief that spectators can't tell the type of medication one is taking. For example, the impact of disclosure in reference to medication-taking behavior may be seen in a 36-year-old female respondent's statement when she said,

> I always take medication on time because I can take it anywhere, since almost everyone knows my HIV serostatus. Even when I am in someone's office I may just mention that, oh! It is time to take my medication. I take out my bottled water and swallow it right there and then. What encourages me is the fact that this very medication is what made me whole again. Even when I am walking down the street no one can pin-point me out that she has AIDS based on physical appearance as used to be the case.

Another theme was value for life. Prioritizing the value for life before embarrassment was made clear by a 54-year-old male soldier, who confidently stressed, "Be it at a wedding ceremony I will openly pull out my medication and swallow it before everyone at the exact appointed time because I am not ashamed of trying to save my life."

A 28-year-old female respondent who regularly took medication on a timely basis regardless of who was around also claimed,

> I am not embarrassed to take my medication while other people are watching because I know that I am just trying to take care of my life. Regardless of where I am, when it is time to take my medication I just get it out and swallow it, regardless of who is watching.

Another female participant also asserted,

> I have no difficulty swallowing medication when others are watching because I take this medicine to save my life. Even if

> someone is sitting right in front of me, she/he will not stop me from swallowing my medication at the appointed time because this is my life and I am going to take care of it.

Perception of AIDS as a global pandemic that affects all humanity—or normalizing the illness—was another theme. As a 41-year-old male participant reported,

> I have no difficulty taking antiretroviral medication on time or because other people are watching due to the fact that, whatever is happening to me is not just for one person. If I choose to hide my condition and refuse to take medication as prescribed, I will only be killing myself. When I realize that the disease has spread around all corners of the world, I take comfort that I am not alone, and it motivates me not to be ashamed.

Numerous participants also revealed that they do not skip taking medication because they believe those around them often do not know the type of medication being taken. A common response was embodied by a 38-year-old male respondent, who said,

> I have no problem taking antiretroviral drugs when others are watching because no one will know the medication I am swallowing is for AIDS. I have never shown any of the visible HIV/AIDS symptoms such as a skin rush or wasting syndrome. People may speculate that I am taking medication to fight off a normal illness like malaria, just like anyone else that does not have HIV.

Carrying Medication and Skipping Taking It

Furthermore, as shown in table 6, when asked if respondents sometimes skip taking medication because it is not with them, the majority (81%) indicated they never and only 19% said they sometimes skip taking medication for this reason. This would indicate that the influence of traveling on medication adherence is also minimal. Nevertheless, unexpected delays emerged as a major theme that influenced skipping taking medication for those who reported adherence failure resulting from traveling without carrying medication. Remembering to carry medication at all times, in contrast, emerged as one of the major themes in explaining why traveling away from home did not influence skipping taking medication.

Many of the 18% who reported sometimes skipping taking medication because of failure to carry it at all times indicated this was due to unexpected delays. For instance, as a 42-year-old male respondent explained,

> I have difficulty taking medication on time because, sometimes I may find that I have gone to look for maize floor [*akawunga*, for wage labor that will buy food] at a certain location and then find I have to go to a different location unexpectedly, which location may be much further than home. In the process, time takes me by surprise. As you may imagine the world in which we live here in Uganda, the one who owes you hides from you. Yet he may be your transportation ticket back home. So you find that time elapses when you are waiting for your pay and you may not get home on time to take medication.

The major theme that emerged for those who did not skip taking medication while traveling was always remembering to take medication along. For example, a 33-year-old male participant stated, "I always put my medicine in the bag first whenever I have to go somewhere. I may forget my shirt, but not my drugs."

Female participants responded in a somewhat similar manner. For example, a 40-year-old female reported, "Whenever I have plans to travel anywhere away from home, my medication goes in my purse first. I always remember to carry my medication with me because I never know if I will delay getting back home."

Social Support and Adherence Behavior

According to Gordillo et al. (1999), individuals with social support are more likely to adhere to medication-taking regiments. Other studies associate the presence of other individuals in the home with medication adherence behavior (Machtinger & Bangsberg, 2008). Social support was included in this study to see if it would give some understanding as to why some individuals fail to adhere to medication regimens and others do not. Based on statistics shown in table 6, social support appears to have some influence on medication adherence behavior because when respondents were asked if they have anyone who supports them in taking medication, the majority (81%) indicated having a person or people who reminded them to take medication. Only 19% said they did not have social support.

Lack of Social Support and Adherence Behavior

One of the interesting findings not dominant in literature was that individuals who reported not having social support referred to self-efficacy and reminder cues as substitutes for social support and hence influential in helping them take medication regularly, even in the absence of social support.

For example, a 55-year-old male soldier who reports a lack of social support but who relies on self-efficacy to take medication affirmed,

> It is my will and in my power to take medication at all times. I do not believe it is anyone else's responsibility to remind me to take medication. I have to be self-supportive because I was also alone on the deathbed, not anyone else. I care about my life too much to depend on anyone for it. I don't need someone else telling me that I need to take medicine when it is I that is interested in life.

A 32-year-old female participant also reported,

> I don't have anyone to support me to take my medication because I live by myself. However, I dedicated myself to follow the doctor's orders from the time I started HAART. I am a strong independent woman. I use my mobile phone alarm clock to remind me of the time to take it.

Or as a 24-year-old male participant put it, "I do not have anyone to remind me to take medicine at work, but I still take it because I know it is my responsibility."

Access to Social Support and Adherence Behavior

Of the 81% who reported access to social support, family or friends were implicated as being supportive in enforcing medication-taking behavior. For example, a 50-year-old male participant illustrated,

> I do not miss taking medication and I always take it on time because there are three people in my household that are on HAART, my wife, one child and myself. We all chose to take it at the same time. It is not easy for all of us three to forget taking the medication. If one forgets, another one reminds them.

Another male participant also asserted,

> I take my medication as prescribed because my wife and children support me to take it. When it is time to take the medication, one of my children or my wife may bring the medication to me with a glass of water. However, even if my family is not around I still remind myself to take the medication.

Medication Representation and Adherence Behavior

Research indicates that medication representation, or beliefs about the effect of medication on a given illness, is influential in determining medication-taking behavior. According to Leventhal and Cameron (1987), patients are more likely to remember taking medication if they know its importance as opposed to those who have doubts about it. As shown in table 6, when asked how respondents feel about the outcome of taking highly active antiretroviral drugs, interestingly, almost all participants (99%) indicated they felt their quality of life would improve if they kept taking medication as prescribed. Only 1% said it would not improve. In other words, almost all respondents were optimistic about a better quality of life outcome if they kept taking highly active antiretroviral drugs, which may explain the high percentages of those who claimed not to skip taking medication (table 6). Clinical immunological gains such as the disappearance of opportunistic illnesses, CD4 cell count, weight gain, and physical energy emerged as the major themes that explain why respondents believed highly active antiretroviral drugs are effective in HIV treatment. For example, as a 28-year-old female participant reported,

> Based on how I feel now, I believe if I continue taking this medication as prescribed my health will continue to improve because this is not how I was. For example, when I went to test for HIV the very first time I was diagnosed with full blown AIDS and came to this facility for treatment. I was started on HAART immediately because I had a severe fever of which I almost died from. I had reached the end of life. However, when I came to this facility the health professionals pampered me and started me on HAART after which my condition improved. This is how I appear today and that is why I believe my quality of life will continue to improve if I comply with treatment regimens.

Or as 33-year-old female respondent put it,

> As I swallow each pill I feel my life is improving because since I started HAART, my health has been getting better. I have put on weight and the health problems that were bothering me such as a chest pain and other opportunistic illnesses cleared.

Males also reported belief in the effectiveness of highly active antiretroviral drugs in treating HIV, given improvements in their health. For example, a 33-year-old male reported,

> If I follow the treatment regimen as prescribed, I believe I will stay healthy because, I cannot tell you otherwise but that, even if I died at this hour I cannot underrate what this medication has done for me. I gained consciousness, my health improved. I feel healed because I am not ill anymore. All health issues stopped as soon as I began HAART and I feel my health will remain good.

Similarly, a 46-year-old male participant who attributed an increase in his CD4 cell count and weight gain to the effect of highly active antiretroviral drugs on HIV also stressed,

> I do not want to skip taking my medication. HAART brought my health to its originality. I had been sick for over seven years. Most

> of the severe illnesses that used to bother me are gone, except for minor fevers and a cough sometimes. Before I started taking this medication, I could not sit down for four hours without sleeping. Currently I can stay awake for twenty-four hours.

Another theme was the respondents' hope for an HIV cure. For example, a 28-year-old female participant asserted,

> I believe that if I keep taking this medication I will be completely healed because compared to what I was before I started HAART, to where I am currently, it is a very big difference. I used to have illnesses like a fever, a cold, and a cough that could not heal. I no longer have those conditions.

A 47-year-old male participant also indicated,

> I really feel that the more I continue taking antiretroviral medication, I will indeed be cured of HIV because the soldiers [CD4 cell count] in my body were only 27 when I started this medication. Six months later they have accumulated to about 190.

In summary, lack of food (59%) and forgetfulness (33%) had the biggest influence on skipping taking medication. Side effects (2%), alcohol use (6%), embarrassment (16%), sleeping through the dose (17%), and not carrying medication (19%) had the least influence on adherence failure. The high percentages of individuals who reported belief in highly active antiretroviral drugs as effective in treating HIV (99%) and who stated they have access to social support (81%) may partially explain the moderate to high percentages of those who claim to comply with medication regimens. Respondents also reported fear of mixing alcohol with medication, being busy, embarrassment, social setting, and unexpected delays when traveling to be influential in skipping taking medication. In contrast, experiences with opportunistic infections, illness and medication representation, doctor communication, trust in the doctor, choosing a convenient time, cues to action, disclosure, value for life, and remembering to carry medication at all times emerged as influential factors in medication adherence (not skipping medication).

Factors That Influence Lifestyle Recommendations Adherence Behavior

The third area investigated in this study was what influences individuals to comply with health providers' lifestyle recommendations. Knowledge of influential lifestyle recommendations adherence factors is essential in the control of the spread of HIV as well as for maximizing benefits from HAART such as medication adherence, which is crucial in developing societies. In studying this area, four indicators were utilized, namely condom use, number of sex partners, alcohol use, and good nutrition. Based on results shown in table 2, despite HAART efforts to promote healthy lifestyles among those under treatment, there appears to be a danger to public health: 40% of the participants reported they did not use condoms regularly, and 38% revealed failure to abstain from alcohol. Respondents complied least with dietary recommendations, with 83% of the individuals reporting failure to access good nutrition. Participants complied most with abstinence from sex or having one sex partner (84% of the respondents). When respondents were asked to explain why they chose not to engage in sex with multiple partners, resentment for people of the opposite sex emerged as an influential factor. Analysis of open-ended responses reveals additional influential factors for adherence to lifestyle recommendations, which include the regular use of condoms, abstinence from alcohol, and having good nutrition. In contrast, poverty, gender power imbalances, and mental health emerged as factors associated with risky sexual behavior, the use of alcohol, and poor nutrition. The following discussion begins with a brief description of lifestyle recommendations, presented in the context of Talcott Parsons's (1951) sick role theory, followed by a discussion of quantitative findings. The final section analyzes qualitative responses to provide a more in-depth portrayal of factors that influence adherence to HAART lifestyle recommendations.

HAART Lifestyle Recommendations

Before proceeding, it is important to understand HAART lifestyle recommendations from Talcott Parsons's perspective. The basic lifestyle recommendations are (a) abstinence or engagement in sex with one sex partner, (b) always using a condom, (c) abstinence from alcohol, and (d) having good nutrition. According to Parsons's sick role theory, illness ought not be self-inflicted—for instance, by engaging in health-risk behaviors. In addition, those affected by illness must have a desire to get well, must seek help from health professionals, and once under treatment must comply with health providers' treatment recommendations. Individuals enrolled in HAART are obligated to comply with the sick role expectations, one of which pertains to safe sex practices. This is because the goal for HAART is not only to prevent HIV from replicating and destroying the CD4 cells after infection but also to control the infection rate. Other lifestyle recommendations include abstinence from alcohol because alcohol is a drug and its chemistry may interfere with HAART results. In addition, the literature reveals that alcohol consumption may contribute to medication adherence failure: its consumption may cause individuals to forget to take medication, and it may lead others to engage in unsafe sexual intercourse. Good nutrition is also recommended for participants. Adequate nutrition is necessary for the functional maintenance of the immune system and to carry out chemical processes within the body (FAO, 2002; Williams & Friedland, 1997). Failure to adhere to these lifestyle recommendations undermines public health efforts to control HIV. Following is a quantitative analysis of adherence to lifestyle recommendations succeeded by a qualitative analysis that explores why individuals on HAART comply or fail to comply with health providers' lifestyle recommendations. As presented in table 2, findings show that only 17% of the respondents report having good nutrition, as opposed to the 83% who do not. Participants comply most with abstinence from sex or having sex with one partner (84% comply), as well as abstinence from alcohol (62%). However, 40% fail to use condoms regularly and 38% fail to abstain from alcohol. In addition to quantitative responses, participants were asked to explain in detail why they complied with or failed to adhere to HAART lifestyle recommendations. The analysis yielded the following results.

There were a number of themes that emerged in the quest for lifestyle recommendations adherence behavior, including resentment of the opposite sex, illness representation, perceived threat of AIDS, birth control, and alcohol representation. In contrast, poverty, gender power imbalances, cultural beliefs, anxiety, addiction, and peer pressure emerged as themes explaining why individuals failed to adhere to HAART lifestyle recommendations. These themes are elaborated in the following few sections.

Adherence to Abstinence or Having Sex With One Partner

One of the goals for HAART is to promote abstinence or having sex with one partner. Table 2 indicates that the vast majority (84%) of the respondents reported abstinence from sex or having one sex partner, with only 16% indicating having multiple (more than one) sex partners. When asked to give reasons for or against engagement in sex with multiple partners, economic need and alcohol use surfaced as major explanatory themes. The major theme that emerged for those who abstained or had sex with one partner was resentment for individuals of the opposite sex.

Reasons for Engaging in Sex With Multiple Partners

Although scholars in developed countries report that one of the effects of HAART is an increase in the prevalence of risky sex behavior because those under therapy perceive themselves as noninfectious as a result of decreased viral load and CD4 cell count, these data indicate that it is not HAART but economic need and alcohol use that induce risky sex behavior (Remien et al., 2007). It is interesting that the theme of economic need was more common among females than males, whereas that of alcohol use was more common among males. For example, a 29-year-old female respondent expressed,

> Since I started highly active antiretroviral drugs, I have had sex with three men. I don't usually want men to bother me. If they keep on disturbing me I give in, sometimes because nature kicks in. After one relationship I may get into another relationship with someone else. I am usually expecting some money from the male partner. When I realize he is not giving me anything I leave him and find another one.

Another female participant driven by economic need to have sex with multiple partners also reported,

> In the last twelve months, I had sex with two men. One of them was a casual partner; the other is my boyfriend whom I think is also having a sexual relationship with another woman. I am still with him regardless of all that because he supports me financially in a significant way, and I think he loves me. I can't get rid of him because he also will not leave me alone. There is no way I can *okwekyanga* [jam or bend out of shape] when he shows me love by giving me money.

Males mostly implicated alcohol use as having an effect on the number of sex partners. For example, as a 33-year-old male participant put it, "Alcohol sometimes makes me sleep with women unexpectedly. I become like a hyena, I may even stop and buy someone to sleep with me. However, even if I am drunk, I still use a condom."

Reasons for Abstinence or Having Sex With One Partner

Both females and males expressed feelings of resentment for the opposite sex as a reason to abstain from sex or to have sex with one sex partner. For example, a 35-year-old female participant who attributed abstinence to disliking males stated,

> I have not slept with any man since I started HAART because I no longer like men. I don't even have a thought of men in my mind to tell you the truth. After knowing my condition, I turned to God and right now it is my God and I.

Another woman who chose abstinence and who attributed not having sex to a resentment for men also asserted,

> I do not want to sleep with men. I already had a lover I lived with at the time I started HAART. However, currently I tell him that, if you feel like having sex, you need to go find another woman because I will not have sex with you. Regardless of if I were to use a condom, from deep down my heart I no longer desire men. I gave up on them.

A male participant who claimed to have had numerous female lovers before, but who has maintained only one girlfriend since HAART initiation, also explained,

> I used to have many girlfriends. Since I started HAART, I have only been with one girlfriend because I feel women lovers give me a heart-burn [*bankeeta*, a slang for something you dislike from deep inside]. I do not like women any more.

Adherence to Condom Use

The use of condoms is relatively new in the Ugandan setting, and it was stressed more after the advent of AIDS. HAART promotes the regular use of condoms for individuals on treatment as a means to control the spread of HIV. To understand why some individuals chose to use condoms regularly as opposed to those who did not, participants were requested to give reasons behind condom use behavior. Gender inequalities, birth control, and cultural beliefs emerged as major themes among those who said they did not use condoms regularly. In contrast, doctor communication, illness representation, perceived threat, and birth control emerged as major themes explaining why individuals used condoms regularly.

Reasons for Failing to Use Condoms

One of the themes that emerged when respondents were asked to explain failure to use condoms regularly was gender power imbalances that situate females in settings where they lack power to decide whether or not to use condoms. This finding is in line with other global studies that portray females in positions powerless to negotiate safe sex (Pulerwitz et al., 2002). For example, a 37-year-old female participant stated,

> I personally believe it is important to use a condom during sexual intercourse, but my husband refuses to use it. I don't know if my husband has other women but he makes the final decision in regards to condom use, and that means that we do not use condoms in our house. He says condoms are too much for him and he does not like them, which I do not understand.

Cultural beliefs pertaining to gender stratification and procreation were also given as reasons for not using condoms. Some respondents reported they did not believe in using condoms with spouses, probably because the institution of marriage values procreation and condoms may hinder pregnancy. It could also be true that males assume their wives are not seeing other men—given the cultural social context that expects females to have only one sex partner, if not to totally abstain from sexual intercourse, a norm that does not usually apply to males. Females in numerous African settings are also perceived as possessions without a voice. These characteristics are detected in a statement of one male respondent, who authoritatively and confidently asserted,

> I do not use a condom with my wife at home because I believe it is only important to use it with outsiders. I will never use a condom at home with my wife. Why would I bring a condom when it is my wife, except if the purpose for using it is to control pregnancy but not safe sex? We do not discuss the condom because it does not concern us, period. However, since I started HAART I have had sexual relationships with two wives. I use a condom with the wife that does not live with me.

Women also portrayed concerns of using condoms with spouses. For example, a 25-year-old female participant stated, "I do not agree that just because I am enrolled in HAART I must use a condom with my husband."

Another female respondent also indicated, "I have no problem following the doctor's orders to take medication. However, I do not agree with some of his advice like when he says I must use a condom even though I am married."

Females who had issues pertaining to using condoms with spouses may have responded in such a manner because they may have felt the need to have children, given the fact that procreation is a cultural value. Belief in procreation is reflected in this statement from one of the male respondents:

> I think it is very important to use a condom but I already had two wives before I started HAART. My wives and I had never heard of the word "condom" until very recently. After being introduced

> to the condom, we tried to use it but it did not go well for us. When I discussed the need to use a condom to both my wives after enrollment in the HAART program, one of them did not agree to use it because she wanted children, which stirred a lot of conflict between us. She accused me of the possibility of having other women saying that I want to use a condom because I do not love her any more. The other wife also did not agree to use a condom. To somewhat balance these differences, we decided to have sex without a condom but only once in two weeks or a month because having sex is a call of nature.

Reasons for Using Condoms Regularly

Among the 60% who reported using condoms regularly, doctor communication was one of the themes that surfaced in explaining regular condom use. For example, a male participant who used condoms regularly stated, "I always use a condom because health providers counseled my wife and I that it is very important to use it. Ever since, I use a condom during sexual intercourse."

Perceived threat of reinfection with a different HIV strain was another emergent theme associated with doctor communication in explaining why some individuals always used condoms. As a 49-year-old male respondent illustrated,

> I was informed by the doctor that there are various types of HIV strains and that not everyone is infected with the same type such that, it is dangerous to mix the different strains through failure to protect oneself. This danger scared me. For that reason alone, even when I pick up someone that is not already HIV positive, I would like to use the plastic [slang for *condom*] so that we do not mix different strains of HIV. So, whenever I sleep with a woman I make sure that I use the condom, 100 percent.

Further indication of how effective HAART education can be in promoting condom use can be seen in a female respondent's statement:

> I don't know if it is necessary for us who have been living with HIV as a married couple to use the plastic [condom] as we have never discussed this issue with a health provider. We have not

> been using a condom because we neither know what a condom is, nor the difference in using it or not. If the health provider says it is necessary, then we shall use it.

In addition to HAART, numerous respondents reported other factors, such as birth control, to be influential in the decision to use a condom. For instance, as a 53-year-old male participant argued,

> I always use a condom because my girlfriend is young and anytime she may become pregnant. Otherwise, if she becomes pregnant, where will I put that child? For that reason I discuss safe sex with my girlfriend and I believe that the man has the power to decide if to use a condom or not. If a woman refuses it, the man should take control because the woman may become pregnant.

Illness representation also explains why some individuals used condoms regularly. This is clear from a 34-year-old male participant's statement:

> I believe that it is important to use a condom because slim [slang for *AIDS*, a term generated from an HIV opportunistic illness referred to as wasting syndrome, which makes infected persons look extremely skinny] is extremely painful such that it is not good to pass it on to any other person. If the other person does not have slim, even if they want to have a child through sexual intercourse, let them first think about the consequences of slim. AIDS really hurts. Because I know how AIDS hurts, I always have condom use on my mind.

Adherence to Abstinence to Alcohol

HAART care providers advise participants to refrain from the use of alcohol because alcohol may foster health-risk behaviors such as engagement in unprotected sexual intercourse or forgetting to take medication (Hardon et al., 2006; Haubrich et al., 1999; Moatti et al., 2000). The results in table 2 indicate that 38% of the respondents reported having used alcohol in the past 6 months. To gain an in-depth understanding of why some individuals on HAART abstain from alcohol use whereas others continue to drink, participants were asked to state reasons for and against alcohol use. Anxiety, addiction, and peer pressure emerged as influential factors for individuals who reported to have used alcohol in the last 6 months, whereas provider communication presented as a major theme in explaining why others abstained from alcohol use.

Reasons for Drinking Alcohol

Many of those who reported having used alcohol in the past 6 months indicated that they were well informed by health providers that HAART does not work well with alcohol. When asked to explain why they choose to drink alcohol despite the health providers' recommendations, anxiety surfaced as an influential factor. Many who referred to anxiety as an impetus for drinking alcohol revealed concerns of poverty as well as fear of dying and leaving their children orphaned. For example, a 28-year-old female respondent stated,

> The doctor told me not to drink. However, anxiety induces my drinking of alcohol. I sometimes say to myself, alcohol will help soothe my emotional pain. If I drink alcohol, I will just fall down and sleep soundly without worries that are usually triggered by questions as to how I am to provide for my children or pay for rent. When I drink I feel relaxed.

Another female respondent also reported,

> I sometimes drink, but not because I like alcohol. I drink to get a temporary escape from worries. However, afterwards I regret as I ask myself why I took it when the doctor advised me not to drink alcohol.

Or as 26-year-old female participant put it, "I drink to make worries disappear so that I can go to sleep."

One of the female respondents also tried to justify alcohol use by arguing,

> I cannot lie to you. A craving for alcohol comes every now and then and I may take some traditional beer. However, alcohol does not make me miss a dose because I begin drinking it in the afternoon

> and I stop earlier than the time I am supposed to take medication. If time is close to that when I am supposed to take medication, I do not drink alcohol, even if it is offered free of charge. Additionally, alcohol does not make me have unprotected sex.

Addiction was another highlighted theme that appears in the explanations of some individuals who drink alcohol. For example, a 44-year-old male with issues of addiction explained,

> Initially I was addicted to alcohol. Currently I may refrain from alcohol use for about three to four months. However, when I start drinking I take it daily. I do not want to crave for alcohol and many times I regret 100 percent, asking myself why I have taken it when the doctors advised me otherwise. During such times it feels like someone who is going to fall into hell.

Another influential factor was peer pressure. Participants reported they knew they should not drink alcohol while under therapy and that they did not want to do it. However, they used alcohol for social reasons. For example, a 40-year-old male participant reported,

> I sometimes take alcohol, often with peers when I am looking for work. I am in the construction business and many times I have to meet with fellow workers waiting for a customer to give me a plan of work. While waiting my peers may give me an offer of alcohol such that I end up drinking despite the fact that the purpose for meeting with my friends was not to drink. However, based on my alcohol use experience, I know how much alcohol to consume.

Another male participant also reported,

> I drink alcohol daily because after work, I am at home where many of my friends come for a social gathering during which alcohol is served. I don't want to drink but my friends usually influence me to drink. The problem is that drinking makes me forget to take my medication.

Females were as likely as males to report the influence of peer pressure on drinking alcohol, despite the efforts of HAART providers to curb its use. As a 34-year-old female stated,

> Health providers advised us not to drink. However, I drink because people offer me drinks at work, usually at a time when I am really thirsty. For example, someone may come and say, give her a very cold beer. If I take the offer I feel guilty afterwards because I know alcohol use is not good for me.

Another female participant also reported, "The doctor told us to refrain from alcohol use because it interferes with the effects of medication. The problem is that I am often influenced by my peers while on the job."

Reasons for Abstaining From Alcohol

Some respondents stated that HAART had an effect on decisions not to drink. Numerous respondents referred to information relayed by health providers against alcohol use. For example, a 37-year-old female respondent stated,

> I used to drink alcohol, but not anymore because the health providers advised us not to drink. In addition, I understood the dangers or consequences of taking alcohol like making me to forget taking my medicine. I also realized that alcohol adds nothing to my life apart from the temporary happiness.

A 22-year-old female respondent also alleged, "I do not drink alcohol because the doctor told me that if I take alcohol while on treatment I am wasting medicine. Because of that, I excused myself of alcohol."

Another theme that emerged in explaining why some individuals refrain from drinking alcohol was alcohol representation. For example, a 52-year-old male respondent who perceived alcohol to cause disease progression explained,

> I used to drink daily, but I completely suspended alcohol use after I realized alcohol had an effect on my health. I felt that the more I used alcohol, the more my health deteriorated. For that

> reason, I stopped alcohol use because I realized that it was a hindrance to the treatment progress. That made me terminate its use.

Adherence to Good Nutrition

HAART health providers also recommend good nutrition for individuals on treatment. Good nutrition is essential for the human body because it boosts the immune system and assists in processes such as digestion. To study the effect of HAART on promoting good nutrition, respondents were asked if they follow the doctor's orders to have a good diet. Findings revealed in table 2 show that 83% of the participants did not follow the health providers' dietary recommendations, as compared to the 17% who did. When they were prompted to explain failure to do so, poverty emerged as the major theme. Many of the respondents expressed feelings of inability to acquire the recommended diet because of economic need. For example, a 29-year-old female respondent reported,

> The doctor says that if you enroll in the HAART program you need to have a good diet. The health providers also inform us that a poor diet makes one feel bad physically. But if you have no money to buy food, what can you do?

A number of male participants also expressed powerlessness to acquire good nutrition. For instance, as indicated by a 43-year-old male respondent,

> I cannot have a good diet because I have no money to buy food. Currently, I am not working because I cannot find a job due to my health condition. My wife is the breadwinner in my household and her job does not pay her well. If I were working, maybe I would be able to access good nutrition as the doctor recommends.

A 36-year-old male respondent also asked,

> Is there any way we can get some assistance with nutrition? This illness needs to affect the rich because without money, even

> treatment with highly active antiretroviral drugs may not be effective. Regardless of the doctor's orders that I must eat well, as a client I also understand that I need good nutrition including dairy products, fruits, meat, and vegetables. However, without money I can't afford a good diet.

As a 33-year-old male respondent reported,

> When I had first started HAART, they used to give us food supplements from international donor organizations and that was very helpful because, most of the people with AIDS begin HAART when we are extremely ill such that we are extremely weak and cannot work. We usually do not have jobs that can support us to buy food. It is sad that as soon as I became somewhat better, food support ended. The problem is that, people with AIDS cannot get jobs that offer a descent pay due to discrimination. It is difficult to have a good diet when you have no money.

In conclusion, participants revealed that failure to adhere to HAART lifestyle recommendations is most influenced by poverty, gender inequality, anxiety, addiction, and peer pressure. Findings also indicate that resentment for people of the opposite sex, birth control, and illness representation were the main factors that influenced individuals not to have sex with multiple partners, to use condoms regularly, and to abstain from alcohol.

The Impact of HAART on Perceived Quality of Life

The impact of HAART on perceived quality of physical and psychological life was the fourth area investigated. Studies—especially those conducted in resource-rich nations—reveal that HAART has been effective in improving the overall quality of life for those under therapy (Lohse et al., 2007; Rowell & Shippy, 2004). However, few studies on the effects of HAART on physical and psychological health for those under therapy in resource-limited nations exist (Bunnell et al., 2006; Jelsma et al., 2005). This study investigates that area, and its findings may help improve the quality of life for those under HAART in developing nations. There were three dummy-coded indicators for investigating this area. They measured 1 for respondent perceives physical health, psychological health, or overall quality of life as somewhat better or much better and 2 for respondent perceives physical health, psychological health, or overall quality of life as the same as or worse than before HAART initiation. The details for these measurements are presented in chapter 3.

Results from this investigation are revealed in table 7; they show that more individuals (91%) reported better physical health since HAART initiation as opposed to those who reported better psychological health (83%). Almost all respondents (94%) indicated improvement in the overall quality of life since HAART initiation. Major themes that explain better physical health include a decrease in opportunistic infections, rise in the CD4 cell count, and weight gain, as well as recovery from immune reconstitution syndrome and side effects. On the other hand, anxiety, hopelessness, and loneliness rooted in

TABLE 7. Perceived quality of life outcomes.

Item	*N*	%
Physical Health		
Somewhat Better or Much Better	64	91.4
The Same or Worse	6	8.6
Total	70	100.0
Psychological Health		
Somewhat Better or Much Better	58	82.9
The Same or Worse	12	17.1
Total	70	100.0
Overall Quality of Life		
Somewhat Better or Much Better	66	94.3
The Same or Worse	4	5.7
Total	70	100.0

Source. Data collected in Uganda, 2007.

poverty and discrimination emerged as major themes in explaining poor psychological health. The discussion of the quality of life for those under HAART that participated in this study begins with an analysis of quantitative responses, followed by that of the qualitative responses as seen below.

Findings as shown in table 7 reveal that HAART has had a major impact on improving the overall quality of life for those under treatment (94% of the participants). The biggest impact of HAART has been on physical health as opposed to psychological health. Statistics in table 7 show that almost all respondents (91%) reported physical health as somewhat better or much better than before HAART initiation. On the other hand, a somewhat smaller percentage (83%) of participants reported that their psychological health was somewhat better or much better since HAART initiation. An analysis of the responses reveals states of physical health, previous experiences with opportunistic illnesses, immune reconstitution syndrome, and side effects as the major explanatory themes. However, anxiety rooted in poverty and perceived threat of disease progression surfaced as themes that explain poor psychological health. The discussion that follows pertains to qualitative analytical findings of the impact of HAART on physical health, followed by that on psychological health.

The Impact of HAART on Physical Health

In this study, participants gave detailed accounts of how HAART transformed their physical health through testimonies that reveal clinical, virological, and immunological gains such as increases in CD4 cell count, decreased opportunistic infections, and weight gain, findings that agree with those conducted in developed societies. Almost all participants reported experiences with opportunistic infections characteristic of AIDS diagnosis. The reader should keep in mind that it is normal for individuals with AIDS to experience multiple opportunistic illnesses concurrently. In that regard, previous experiences with opportunistic infections were one of the dominant themes in rating physical health as participants compared the current states of their health to those before HAART.

In order to fully grasp the meaning of HAART to participants in the discussion of quality of life below, it is important to realize that palliative care is almost nonexistent in Uganda. In that regard, respondents who indicated that HAART has improved their physical health described experiences with opportunistic infections before HAART as characterized by excruciating, agonizing pain. Their distress was relayed through their body language, gestures, voice tones, and verbal expressions in a depth that no English words could express. In addition to herpes zoster, participants revealed experiences with skin rashes, sores from the mouth down to the esophagus and into the stomach, weight loss, vivid dreams, weakness, and lack of appetite as manifested in the most severe way. With the advent of highly active antiretroviral drugs and medication adherence, these illnesses improved or the patients were healed. Below is a glimpse of how respondents described manifestations of opportunistic illnesses in the absence of palliative care as well as testimonies in reference to the impact of HAART on health. The first testimony is that of a 45-year-old male participant, who stated,

> Before I started HAART, I lived in so much physical pain that if poison was in my reach, I would have taken my life, and there were times when I pleaded to my relatives to bring me poison so that I could end it all. For example, when *kisipi* [slang for herpes zoster] hit me I was in severe pain, it hurt me to the extreme. I used to move around in a towel, for two weeks. It is now five years since kisipi hit me, and although with HAART I feel healed from it, I am still experiencing its impact.

The impact of HAART in improving physical health is also detected in a 45-year-old female respondent's testimony.

> My health is somehow good because I was in a severe condition. I used to have sores in my mouth down to the esophagus and stomach. At the same time I constantly experienced skin rush, nausea, fever and a headache for which I continuously took panadol and whatever pill I thought would be of help, but nothing improved these health conditions. I never knew my skin was like canvas

> because I used to scratch and scratch and scratch. However, it is two months since I started HAART and I have not scratched since. I was also healed of the fever and the headache.

Likewise, a 37-year-old male participant who had been on therapy for more than 6 months testified,

> My overall health is good because six months can go by without becoming sick, except for a cough or cold. Before I started this medication, I used to have piercing pain in the chest and a constant fever. If I tried to do manual work, I would get a piercing pain in the chest after which I would start panting for air and coughing. However, since I started taking highly active antiretroviral drugs, I feel good physically.

Some of the respondents reported experiences with chronic sexually transmitted infections, which disappeared when they began taking highly active antiretroviral drugs. For instance, as a 29-year-old female participant remarked,

> Before I started taking highly active antiretroviral drugs, I was frequently affected by sexually transmitted diseases and they had taken away all my peace. In addition, I always had fever and I was so weak. Since I began taking this medication, I don't have most of these conditions and I have energy.

Another theme that emerged as evidence for the impact of HAART on physical health was the immune reconstitution syndrome. Although HAART leads to improvements in the quality of health in the long run, the initial impact may be deterioration of health, as revealed by some respondents who reported experiences with immune reconstitution syndrome. Immune reconstitution syndrome refers to a cluster of opportunistic illnesses that emerge during treatment when the CD4 cells begin to increase and to fight against latent opportunistic illness–causing agents that may exist within the body before an individual takes highly active antiretroviral drugs. That is, one of the purposes of highly active antiretroviral therapy is to enable reconstitution or repair of the immune system, which leads to an increase in the CD4 cells, whose function is to fight off infections.

However, in some people the reconstitution of the immune system may trigger the onset of opportunistic illness manifestations, whose agents may have been latent before HAART initiation. Although immune reconstitution syndrome often lasts only for a few weeks or months with continued use of highly active antiretroviral drugs, some of the illnesses may become severe before one's physical health begins to improve (Cheonis, 2005). Some of the participants in this study reported a deterioration of health soon after HAART initiation, attributable to the immune reconstitution syndrome. A few participants who had been on therapy for less than 6 months and were still experiencing this syndrome reported poor health. Many of the respondents who had been on treatment for more than 6 months and who reported physical health as somewhat better or much better than before HAART recalled experiences with immune reconstitution syndrome. As a 23-year-old female respondent exclaimed,

> As soon as I started taking highly active antiretroviral drugs, it appeared like the drugs unraveled every illness in my body, exposing every hidden health condition that had ever existed in my system. For example, I developed a terrible skin rash manifested in the most extreme pain. However, the doctor had informed me about getting side effects and he had encouraged me to be strong...In my case, it took three months to recover from these illnesses before I began feeling good.

Another respondent also stated,

> Soon after beginning to take highly active antiretroviral drugs, I developed a severe pounding headache. It would pound, and pound, and pound. At the same time, water would flow from my head such that I would tie a headscarf around it, but within six minutes, it was dripping wet. As I continued taking highly active antiretroviral drugs, everything was healed. I feel good today.

Side effects were another theme that emerged as participants explained the impact of HAART on physical health. Side effects normally affect those who have been on treatment for less than 6 months. Some of the side effects mentioned included numbness in the limbs, fever, skin rush, chest pain, and vivid dreams. Participants who had been on HAART for more than 6 months testified that their physical health was better or much better than before because they had been healed of side effects. As a 56-year-old-male respondent recalled,

> When I first took the highly active antiretroviral drugs, I frequently had vivid dreams, I think it was the medicine. This would go on every day, all night or as long I lay down sleeping. However, as I continued to take highly active antiretroviral drugs, the vivid dreams decreased in number, until when they totally stopped. I have no trouble sleeping at the moment as used to be the case when I had vivid dreams.

However, a number of participants who had been on therapy for less than 6 months reported better physical health, though they had not yet reached a point where they could say their physical health was very good because of side effects. As explained by a 50-year-old male soldier who had been on therapy for 4 months,

> Compared to how I was before HAART, I feel I am beginning to get some energy. However, after beginning therapy I developed numbness in my foot. I cannot use my right foot to walk if I am not wearing boots. My right arm is also paralyzed and it shakes occasionally, but I would say that although my health is not excellent, it is much better than before I started HAART.

A 27-year-old female participant also indicated,

> Before I started taking this medication, I was in such a bad state. I used to be extremely skinny. I had sores running from my mouth, down the esophagus to the stomach. It is about four months now and I no longer experience those illnesses. However, I can't say that I feel very good because, even if I don't have the fever, my legs began to swell when I began taking this medication, they feel numb and hurt at the bottom.

Another female participant who had been on HAART for 5 months also indicated,

> Since I started taking highly active antiretroviral drugs, there is a difference in my physical health because am no longer constantly sick as before. However, I usually get a fever and a cold. Those are my illnesses. I also can't carry firewood or fetch water. Sometimes I feel weak.

Males who had been on treatment for less than 6 months also revealed that although their health was better, they still experienced a few health conditions. As detected in one of the statements made by a 34-year-old male participant,

> I have been on treatment for about one month, but I am still sickly. I experience severe pain mainly in the lower limbs where I constantly feel a burning sensation. My health sometimes limits my bending and lifting light objects. Sometimes my health limits my dressing and bathing.

Among the few respondents who indicated physical health to have remained the same as or worse than before HAART initiation was a 36-year-old female who reported, "At times I feel very discouraged because, since I started treatment, I am not sure if my physical health is improving. Probably I feel it is about the same because I still feel bad."

In summary, the vast majority of respondents (91%) reported HAART had been largely effective in improving physical health. However, although numerous participants—especially those who had been on treatment for less than 6 months—revealed that their physical health was somewhat better than before, they reported they were not completely well as a result of experiences with immune reconstitution syndrome or side effects or, as some reported, they had not been totally healed of opportunistic infections. Very few respondents reported physical health as being the same as or worse than before HAART initiation.

The Impact of HAART on Psychological Health

Similarly, although the percentage is somewhat smaller than that of those who reported improvements in physical health (91%), the vast majority (83%) of respondents reported improvements in psychological health.

The major themes that resounded in explaining psychological states of health include anxiety, fear, and loneliness, which participants revealed as rooted in poverty, discrimination, and feelings of helplessness to care for family. The reduced impact of HAART on psychological versus physical health may be because these programs do not provide medical mental health services; in addition, they do not address the underlying causes of psychological distress embedded in the socioeconomic contexts, such as poverty and discrimination, as may be the case in developed nations. For instance, a 50-year-old female participant expressed anxiety because of her poverty by stating,

> I don't worry about my physical health, but I worry because of poverty because after my husband died I became the man in the household [breadwinner], and at the same time I remained the mother who provides care for my children, yet I do not have a job. Sometimes I ask myself how I will be able to put my children through school. I may also ask myself that, if I get extremely sick, who will take care of me or who will raise them?

A significant number of male participants also referred to anxiety as a result of poverty and expressed concerns for not being able to care for their family. For example, a 39-year-old male respondent indicated,

> Poverty is the source of my worries not AIDS because we do have antiretroviral medication such that, I feel I can even live another 50 years. However, I worry about my job and the money I don't have. Now I am gambling for money to take care of my children.

A 42-year-old male also expressed concerns about lack of food by stating,

> Health providers recommend that we remain worry free. However, I sometimes feel anxious because of the economy. What worries me most is lack of food. If I have food to eat such that I am able to take medication as prescribed, I am at peace. The only time I am scared is when I fail to adhere to the doctor's orders because I don't have food to eat.

Others referred to concerns for unemployment as a source of anxiety. For example, a 40-year-old male explained,

> My physical health is better, but most of the time I am sad because I am not working. As a man if you have no money in your pocket, it is worrisome and it makes you feel hopeless. I usually ask myself that in reality if I die today, what will happen to my daughter? I have nothing to think of at the moment that I can leave for her for financial support.

Some participants associated poverty with loneliness or lack of social-economic support. As indicated by a male respondent,

> Poverty and loneliness is what worries me. I may begin thinking; my old man [father] just left us yesterday [died], which makes me feel lonely. Perceiving my health, I realize it has also narrowed my territory. Then I become restless because of those conditions. Most of the time I may take time to be silent, reflect on my life and try to imagine where the world is taking me. There are times when I feel hopeless...The only time I am at peace and happy is when I have some money to provide for my family, and I can see my children playing and laughing because they have had something to eat. However, if I am in a crashing situation as is usually the case, I feel sad in my heart and sometimes so afraid because of my health and what would become of my children without me.

Discrimination was another theme that surfaced as participants discussed their psychological health. For example, a 35-year-old male respondent explained,

> I don't worry about health anymore because I have highly active antiretroviral drugs that have made me well. However, I worry about employment. The problem is that, when people find out that one has AIDS, they discriminate against that person from work such that it would be difficult for anyone to give him/her a job. The employer may say, I cannot hire someone that has the insect [HIV]. It is difficult for us who have HIV to understand why employers feel that way because if the employer gives me a job, I

> will do it well for them. If I can get a job that will provide something to eat and drink, I would be happy and at peace.

Other job-related concerns were also mentioned as reasons for anxiety. For instance, a 43-year-old male soldier explained,

> Anxiety usually arises from duty related issues. I am a soldier. I may go to work one day and my superiors may inform me that I have been stationed somewhere on the front line when my health status is not good for conditions there. That is when I become extremely anxious and I begin to worry, but not because of having AIDS.

Some of the respondents referred to the perceived threat of AIDS as a source of anxiety, sadness, and loneliness. This is detected in a statement made by a 43-year-old male respondent, who reported,

> Sometimes I am so afraid that I tremble, especially after I look at a fellow HIV patient because I start wondering if I am about to reach that stage. There was a time when I came here for treatment and saw a patient with a condition that I had never seen in my life. By just looking at him, I felt sicker. After a few minutes of looking at my fellow patient, I told the nurse that I was going home without treatment because I could not bear the fear any more.

The same respondent also related another scenario:

> One time I had just boarded a taxi [it looks like a minibus that seats about 15 passengers], but at the next stop someone with AIDS also boarded the same taxi. The patient appeared to be in such a bad shape and he was so skinny. Looking at his condition, I told the taxi driver that I forgot something and that I needed to get off the taxi at the next stop. I did that to avoid being on the same taxi with my fellow patient because it was difficult to travel with him.

Numerous respondents also expressed fears of socializing with others, and they often pointed to stigma as an impediment to mixing with others. As one of the female respondents indicated, "This illness hinders me from socializing with family and friends. I have specific places that I do not want to go because I feel I will run into people who will discover I have AIDS."

Another female participant also stated,

> My health stops me from socializing because I feel I don't fit in with people I perceive to be healthy. For example, my lips are red because of an HIV related health condition, which is a sign that others may see and immediately realize that I have AIDS. The reddening of my lips has taken my peace away. Sometimes I want to socialize or travel but I say to myself that, eh! there will be a lot of people and they may notice my health condition. That alone hinders me from socializing with others making me feel extremely lonely.

Some of the respondents who reported better psychological health indicated that health providers advised them not to worry, which functioned as an antidote for anxiety. For example, a female respondent who related to health provider communication and religion as antidotes for anxiety explained,

> I don't worry anymore. For one thing I have been counseled. Another thing is that, I believe in God who gives me peace of mind. I used to feel sad and lonely, but not after I started HAART. The Bible is also my comfort. It tells me how to overcome anxiety. I am not afraid of my health outcome anymore.

However, despite health providers' recommendations to refrain from anxiety, some participants reported that anxiety was difficult to overcome. This is revealed in a statement given by a 46-year-old male:

> My counselors say not to worry as it cannot change any situation. In that case, I often dismiss worries. However, soon after I do that, I snap back into thinking for example, that I am an adult obligated to take care of my children and myself. In addition, I realize that my clan or relatives know that I am sick and cannot work. Although they could help me with financial support, they don't care because they have the assumption that I will die tomorrow. Then I may think, if I ceased to exist today, with whom will I leave my children? That thought brings tears to eyes. Additionally, sometimes I have no money, yet my children need school fees and at the same time I have to pay for my rent. I become even more hopeless when I realize I do not own a home, and I don't have

> a job that would enable me to build a home for my family such that at least if I die, they will have a place to stay. Such thoughts generate anxiety. However, I have confidence in God as my hope because I believe that He knows my situation and He cares.

In conclusion, an overwhelming majority (94%) agreed that HAART has had a big impact on improving their overall quality of life. The biggest impact of HAART was on physical health as opposed to psychological health, with 91% of the respondents reporting better physical health since HAART initiation. Many of the participants reported a decrease in opportunistic infections and increase in CD4 count, as well as recovery from immune reconstitution syndrome. The percentage (83%) of those who reported psychological health as somewhat or much better than before HAART was somewhat smaller than that (91%) of those who reported physical health as somewhat or much better. Anxiety, hopelessness, and loneliness rooted in poverty and discrimination emerged as major themes in explaining poor psychological health. HAART programs do not address these issues, which may explain why the impact of HAART on psychological health has been less than that on physical health.

Chapter 5

Conclusion

HAART Adherence Behavior

In reviewing the distribution patterns of HAART adherence behavior by gender, age, and education level, it was found that the percentage (49%) of participants who did not always take medication on time is about the same as that (51%) of those who always took medication on time. Likewise, almost half (41%) of the respondents reported that they sometimes skipped taking medication. In addition, 82% of the respondents indicated they did not always follow health providers' advice to have good nutrition, 40% did not always use a condom, and about 38% failed to abstain from alcohol. These findings should be taken seriously, especially given the dangers of suboptimal adherence leading to the formation of a transmissible drug-resistant HIV strain and the potential increase in HIV infection rate, all of which undermines the effects of HAART.

Findings also reveal that females and the less educated were more likely to skip taking medication as compared to other population groups. This could be attributed to economic need, which may hinder access to food necessary to take medication. That is, highly active antiretroviral drugs are free, but health providers require that some medication be taken on a full stomach, and individuals are accountable for their food supply. Gender-constructed roles that deny women a good education and employment opportunities usually position females low in the social stratification system whereby they often earn less than males, which may make them more susceptible to a lack of food as compared to males (Kerbo, 2003). Likewise, education acts as a key to positioning in the social stratification system because lack of education limits employment opportunities. Less educated individuals, if employed, often acquire low-paying jobs as compared to those with more education (Mirowsky, Ross, & Reynolds, 2000). Because females and less educated individuals are less likely to access the food necessary to take medication as required, these population groups are also more likely to skip taking medication as compared to males and the more educated groups, which are often positioned at the top of the social stratification system.

However, males and more educated individuals were more likely to take medication late as compared to females and the less educated individuals. This could be attributed to the fact that males and more educated individuals have a higher probability of working outside of the home as compared to females and the less educated, which makes them more likely to forget it is time to take medication if they are busy at work or to forget to carry it to the workplace. In many parts of the developing world such as Uganda, females often work in homes raising children and performing other domestic tasks. Working from home may have made it more feasible for females than males to take medication on time.

Findings also revealed that less educated individuals and females were less likely to use condoms than males and the more educated. Individuals on HAART in Uganda have free access to condoms. In that regard, one would question why these population groups failed to use condoms. One of the reasons could be partially attributed to social positioning. As Weiss and Lonnquist (2003) reveal, population groups at the bottom of the social stratification system—such as females and the less educated—are more likely to reject healthy lifestyles. Some scholars have argued that less educated individuals are less likely to engage in proven healthy behaviors because lack of education diminishes their sense of personal or social control over their lives and that these population groups have less social support as compared to the more educated (Mirowsky et al., 2000). Cultural beliefs may also partially explain why females utilized condoms less than males. For example, in Uganda as in many African patriarchal societies, people generally believe females are inferior to males, which creates a lack of control for females to negotiate safe sex (Pulerwitz et al., 2002). This theory is supported in this study: numerous females expressed feelings of powerlessness in taking control over the issue of using condoms during sexual intercourse.

Males and more educated individuals were more likely to engage in sex with multiple partners and to drink alcohol as compared to females and those with no or primary education. This could also be explained by social positioning in that males and more educated individuals possess more economic power than their counterparts, meaning that they are more likely to be able to afford to engage in such behavior.

Furthermore, findings in this study reveal that individuals over age 30 used condoms less than those of ages 20 to 29. This could be because individuals over age 30 are more likely to engage in monogamous relationships that carry a higher degree of trust for one another as compared to those between ages 20 to 29, who may still be searching for life partners. Another finding was that respondents between ages 20 to 29 reported using alcohol about twice as often as those over age 30.

Although some of the findings were statistically insignificant, these results are consistent with the literature (e.g., Mirowsky et al., 2000; Pulerwitz et al., 2002). One of the reasons why some of the results were insignificant may pertain to the fact that the sample in this study was small ($N = 70$). Additionally, convenience sampling was utilized to select participants, so the sample was not representative of the entire population on HAART in Uganda from which it was drawn.

ANTIRETROVIRAL DRUG ADHERENCE BEHAVIOR INFLUENTIAL FACTORS

The results of the study revealed that some of the population groups under study did not adhere to treatment regimens. The second investigation area was concerned with why some individuals did not take medication as prescribed as opposed to those who did. Results revealed that lack of food was a major influential factor in skipping taking medication. One of the reasons why lack of food was reported to be a key obstacle to medication adherence may be the impact of HIV/AIDS on the social and economic well-being of the family. Often individuals affected by AIDS are the breadwinners, yet they may find themselves without employment because of illness or discrimination resulting from the stigma attached to HIV. Unemployment may lead to economic insecurity, poverty, and hence lack of resources to buy food necessary to take medication regularly (FAO, 2008). The median income for the participants in this study was $28 (U.S.) per month, which means that many of the respondents earned less than $1 a day. It is important to note that participants were between ages 18 and 64, and a large percentage of them may have had children who shared the meager economic resources. Lack of sufficient income is an obstacle to food access, which may have influenced skipping taking medication.

Another finding was that, unlike in studies conducted in developed nations, side effects had the least influence on skipping taking medication. This could be attributed to medication representation, trust and confidence in health providers, and the presence of social support. Numerous respondents did show courage to take medication in the midst of side effects because they strongly believed highly active antiretroviral drugs were effective in treating HIV. Almost all participants (99%) believed that the quality of life improves if one takes medication regularly. In addition, participants expressed confidence in the health providers and often mentioned that they trusted their counsel that side effects would be temporary, which motivated their continual intake of medications regardless of side effects.

This study also found that embarrassment, sleeping through the dose, and not carrying medication had a somewhat minimal impact on skipping taking medication. The minimal impact may be explained by access to social support and previous experiences with opportunistic illnesses. Over three quarters (81%) of the participants reported that they had someone who reminded them to take medication. However, respondents who reported not having social support revealed that memories of physical suffering from opportunistic illnesses motivated them to take medication as prescribed.

HAART Lifestyle Adherence Behavior Influential Factors

The third investigated area was concerned with what influences compliance or noncompliance with lifestyle recommendations. Respondents revealed that they were well informed by health professionals about the dangers that may arise from failure to adhere to HAART lifestyle recommendations, such as safe sex, abstinence from alcohol, and good nutrition. Yet some individuals chose noncompliance. The main reasons for noncompliance were gender power imbalances, cultural beliefs, and economic need. For instance, participants indicated that they had free access to condoms; however, females expressed feelings of helplessness to negotiate safe sex because they believed males possessed the power to decide whether to use condoms or not. Females were also more likely than males to report engagement in sex with multiple partners because of economic need. These findings are in line with other studies, which have revealed that females often engage in sex with multiple partners for material gains such as money, housing, food, or education (Rieker & Bird, 2000). This behavior may also be attributed to gender-constructed roles that position females in the lower social strata, often making them more economically insecure than males.

Another finding was that although cultural beliefs are often deeply embedded in the mosaic of social contexts, psychological forces had potential to break through cultural barriers to change sexual behavior. For instance, polygamy is generally tolerated in many African settings that encourage procreation, as in Uganda. However, individuals who abstained from sex or had sex with one partner reported that resentment toward the opposite sex influenced their decisions to refrain from having sex with multiple partners.

The Impact of HAART on Perceived Quality of Life

The fourth investigated area explored individuals' perceptions on health outcomes. As revealed earlier, the vast majority (94%) of the participants reported improvements in overall quality of life since HAART initiation. HAART was perceived as very effective in improving physical health, with respondents testifying of such clinical gains as control of opportunistic illnesses, increased CD4 cell count, weight gain, and acquisition of physical energy. Even many of those who had been on therapy for less than 6 months and who were still experiencing manifestations of side effects and immune reconstitution syndrome perceived their health as better than before HAART initiation. Very few individuals (6%) perceived health as the same as or worse than before HAART. Respondents attributed improvements in physical health to highly active antiretroviral drugs.

In contrast, the effects of HAART on perceived psychological health were reported to be somewhat less than those reported on perceived physical health. Numerous respondents expressed feelings of anxiety, fear, and loneliness often resulting from concerns for poverty, discrimination, feelings of helplessness to care for family, and fear of leaving children orphaned without financial security in case of their own death. HAART may have had less impact on psychological health because these programs neither provide medical treatment for mental health nor address underlying causes of psychological distress—such as poverty and discrimination, which are often embedded in the social or economic contexts of developing societies such as Uganda.

Theoretical Implications

Discussed in chapter 2 were relevant existing psychosocial and public health theories of adherence behavior. At that point, I noted that none of the existing theories fully explain HAART adherence behavior in low-income nations, which creates a need for a theory that attempts to exhaustively explain such behavior in these settings.

The HBM is most applicable to this study, but it is limited in that it only addresses the cognitive aspects of adherence behavior while understating the sociological. For example, according to the HBM, individuals are more likely to take medication as prescribed if they perceive illness to be serious, an assertion that is supported in this study. In addition, the HBM also states that individuals are more likely to take medication as prescribed if they perceive that they will benefit from taking the drugs. This is also supported in this study because the majority (99%) of the respondents believed that quality of life improves with the regular intake of highly active antiretroviral drugs. The HBM further indicates that individuals are more likely to take medication as prescribed if perceived barriers (such as lack of food and side effects) do not overwhelm them. This last statement is also partially borne out in this study. For example, respondents who sometimes skipped taking medication reported lack of food to be an overwhelming obstacle in taking medication regularly. However, although side effects may also be perceived as an obstacle to medication intake, findings in this study reveal that they had almost no impact on skipping taking medication, an indication that the HBM does not fully explain HAART adherence behavior.

A more comprehensive explanation of medication adherence behavior may require the integration of the HBM with other psychosocial theories, such as the social support model, which may partially explain why side effects in this study did not influence failure to take medication as prescribed. For instance, the majority (81%) of respondents indicated that they had family or friends who supported them in taking medication. Scholars have noted that loving, affectionate relationships with kin and friends often have the potential to regulate one's thoughts, feelings, and behavior or to raise one's self-efficacy by strengthening coping skills (Redding et al., 2000). In that regard, family and friends may have played a role in enhancing adherence to medication-taking regimens for those who were experiencing side effects manifestation.

Another flaw in the HBM is that it assumes HAART adherence behavior to be volitional, whereas participants in this study revealed the existence of obstacles over which they had no control that made it difficult to comply with the health providers' treatment regimens. For instance, respondents expressed feelings of helplessness to take drugs regularly because they lacked economic power to buy food necessary to take medication. This was also true in instances in which females reported a desire to use condoms but felt powerless to negotiate safe sex because they believed males had the power to decide whether to use condoms or not. This flaw in the HBM may be rectified by drawing from Robert Connell's (1987) theory of gender power, which may explain the role of gender power inequalities in shaping HAART adherence behavior. The gender power theory explains variance in risky sexual behaviors rooted in social contexts where cultural beliefs and values may render females powerless to control their sex behaviors, such as the regular use of condoms.

Overall, a challenge remains for scholars to formulate an integrated theory that fully explains HAART adherence behavior in low-income nations. Although the HBM helps to explain much of this behavior, it is limited because it assumes health behavior to be volitional, which undermines influential factors embedded in the social, economic, and cultural contexts, especially as seen in Uganda and other low-income nations. A more effective, integrated theory for explaining HAART adherence behavior in these settings may combine the HBM, the social support model, and the theory of gender power.

Implications for Practice

Widespread access to HAART in low-income regions is increasing, but HIV/AIDS therapy in this area is still in its infancy. Nevertheless, future efficient provision of HAART-related services might require that researchers and providers learn from the operation of existing centers. Based on the results in this study, individuals currently enrolled in HAART-providing programs in Uganda need more comprehensive care. For instance, in chapter 4, I discussed the dilemma of an obligation to adhere to HAART regimens in the midst of poverty. Many of the respondents indicated that they sometimes skip taking medication because of lack of food, do not always have good nutrition, or sometimes engage in sex with multiple partners as a result of economic need. Given the dangers pertaining to suboptimal adherence and the potential increase in HIV infection rate, HAART-providing centers need to incorporate nutritional and economic support services. It is important, however, to realize that an endeavor to provide nutritional support may be costly given the millions of people receiving free HAART in low-income nations. In that regard, access to nutritional support may be profitably targeted to individuals who need these services the most, such as those who have been in treatment for 6 months or less.

In other words, HAART initiation in Uganda strictly follows the WHO guidelines whereby those enrolled must be in the last stages of the disease, often characterized by severe outbreaks of opportunistic illnesses. After HAART initiation, the restoration of the immune system's function may take about 6 months before it can effectively fight off opportunistic infections. Nutritional support is especially needed during the first 6 months: individuals under therapy may be sickly because of opportunistic illnesses or the immune reconstitution syndrome such that they are sometimes unable to work and thus to access food due as a result of financial constraints. As the quality of life improves, follow-up services—helping individuals acquire employment, for instance—may be provided with a goal to wean them off nutritional support. At the same time, long-term strategies such as those that address issues of stigma and discrimination should also be devised. For example, numerous respondents in this study portrayed a desire to work but could not find employment because of discrimination. In that regard, it may be necessary for government at the national level to enact equal opportunity employment laws that would constrain employers and fellow employees from discriminating against those with HIV.

Furthermore, in order to increase the effects of HAART on psychological health, it is necessary to provide access to mental health medical treatment for such conditions as anxiety and addiction to alcohol. Findings in this study reveal that HAART has had less of an impact on improving psychological health than on physical health. Numerous respondents expressed feelings of anxiety, most of which were rooted in poverty. Although treated with medication in developed nations, anxiety in many of the developing countries (including Uganda) is not medically treated because of financial constraints. Some of the participants reported using alcohol as an antidote for anxiety. Others indicated addiction as the reason why they used alcohol. Alcohol consumption poses the danger of interfering with HAART treatment outcomes. Individuals who take alcohol may forget to take medication or engage in risky sexual behaviors such as failure to use a condom or engaging in sex with multiple partners, which undermine the effects of HAART on those affected. Many of the respondents expressed feelings of guilt after drinking alcohol, which shows that medicine as an alternative to alcohol in the treatment of anxiety may be preferred.

There is also a need for long-term goals. Attempting to normalize HIV/AIDS through nationwide education programs that may utilize media in an endeavor to reduce stigma should be a primary goal. Employers should also be educated on how to support individuals with HIV. Sensitizing employees about the issues of AIDS and the rights of those with HIV in the workplace—and holding employees who violate these rights accountable—could do this. The long-term effects of such education could help those infected with the virus to feel more at ease in public settings so that they may be less embarrassed to take medication as required. In the short run, individuals on therapy may be counseled and encouraged to disclose their HIV serostatus to those around them—friends, family members, and fellow employees—who may be present when they are taking medication. As revealed in chapter 4, individuals who reported taking medication regularly indicated that they did so because they were not ashamed to take it among individuals to whom they had disclosed.

Future Research

Since the treatment's discovery in 1996, some studies on HAART adherence behavior and its impact on the quality of life for those with

HIV/AIDS have been conducted both in developed and developing nations. However, many of these studies are cross-sectional. Therefore, there is a need for longitudinal studies that examine this area, especially in low-income nations that have been affected the most by the disease. That is, unlike cross-sectional studies that examine such phenomenon at one point in time, longitudinal studies may reveal changes in adherence behavior and quality of life over time. A few longitudinal studies conducted in high-income nations may exist. However, although crucial, studies that show long-term effects of HAART on those affected in low-income nations are scarce. It is important to note that unlike in the United States, where HAART has been available to the wider community since 1996, access to HAART for the public in Uganda is a recent phenomenon that began in 2004. As table 1 reveals, over half (53%) of the respondents in this study had been on HAART for 1 year or less, and only 18% reported enrollment in HAART before 2003.

Further still, more studies with larger and more representative samples are also necessary to effectively isolate differences in adherence behavior and the impact of HAART on the quality of life by demographic characteristics. As mentioned earlier, although some of the findings in this study were consistent with the literature, they were insignificant. This could have been partially because the sample was small (70), selected using convenience sampling, and therefore unrepresentative. For example, the median income of the respondents was $28, which means that a large number of participants were earning less than $1 a day. In addition, only 13% of the respondents were Muslim as compared to the 87% who were Christian. Hence, results in this study excluded the more affluent individuals, and they did not explain the effects of religion on adherence behavior. Studies that take a quantitative approach may enrich qualitative studies of this nature. Some of the advantages of quantitative studies are that they make the study of large samples feasible, allow the use of advanced social statistical techniques, and present findings that may be generalized if the sample is selected at random.

Correspondingly, future research may also benefit from quantitative studies generated from medical records instead of using self-reported data, which is often used in studies of this nature. Quantitative studies from medical records could take a longitudinal approach, possibly revealing changes pertaining to the impact of HAART on physical health over time—say in reference to levels of increase in CD4 cell counts and viral loads, as well as frequency and duration of specific opportunistic illnesses, side effects, or immune reconstitution syndrome after HAART initiation. Other quantitative studies from medical records that may increase knowledge are those that measure the effects of nutritional support on improvements in physical and psychological health of those under HAART.

Moreover, this study was conducted in areas around the capital city of Uganda. There is a need for qualitative and quantitative studies conducted not only in the urban but also in rural areas across Uganda and other developing countries, some studies of which may facilitate a comparative meta-analysis of the findings in search for a deeper understanding of adherence behavior and quality of life for those on HAART in low-income nations.

It is also important to note that there is a need for developing and testing a comprehensive theory that would explain HAART adherence behavior across demographic characteristics in low-income nations such as Uganda. As indicated earlier in this chapter, existing theories do not fully explain such behavior.

In conclusion, this volume reveals new information pertaining to HAART adherence behavior in Uganda, knowledge that may enrich the body of literature. In addition, public health, policy makers, and scholars may also benefit from these findings. For instance, it has been revealed that about half of the individuals on HAART do not adhere to medication-taking regimens. Suboptimal medication adherence poses such dangers as the development of a drug-resistant HIV strain. Population groups facing a high risk of skipping taking medication—for instance, females and the less educated—have been identified. Males and the more educated have been identified in reference to being at the highest risk for failing to have sex with only one partner or abstaining from alcohol use. Influential factors for adherence, such as economic need, stigma, and gender power imbalances, have also been highlighted. Although it has been revealed that the majority of respondents perceived quality of life as somewhat or much better than before HAART initiation, findings show that there is a need to increase HAART effectiveness through the provision of more comprehensive care, including services such as nutritional support and mental treatment. This study also reveals a need for a more integrated theory to explain HAART adherence behavior, especially in low-income nations such as Uganda.

References

360: The Positive Care Center at UCSF. (2008). Welcome to 360: The Positive Care Center at UCSF. University of California, San Francisco. Retrieved from http://www.positivehealth.ucsf.edu/.

Abah, S. J., Addo, E., Adjei, P. C., Arhin, P., Barami, A. A. S., Byarugaba, M. A., … Zeeman, H. (2005). There's hope: Early observations of ARV drugs treatment roll out in South Africa. *Essential Drugs Monitor, 34*, 16–17.

AIDS*info*. (2008). HIV and its treatment: Recommended HIV treatment regimens. Washington, DC: U.S. Department of Health and Human Services. Retrieved from http://aidsinfo.nih.gov/Guidelines/Default.aspx?MenuItem=Guidelines.

AIDS InfoNet. (2011). What is antiretroviral therapy? Arroyo Seco, NM: New Mexico AIDS Education and Training Center, University of New Mexico Health Science Center. Retrieved from http://www.aidsinfonet.org/fact_sheets/view/403.

AIDS Services of North Texas. (2007). Creating healthier futures for North Texans living with HIV/AIDS. Plano, TX. Retrieved from http://www.healthntx.org/services/hiv_aids_services.html.

The AIDS Support Organization (TASO). 2006. *TASO Uganda Limited: 2005 Annual Report*. Kampala, Uganda: Author.

Aliouat-Denis, C. (2008). Pneumocystis species, co-evolution and pathogenic power. *Infection, Genetics & Evolution, 8*(5), 708–726.

Altice, F. L., Smith-Rohrberg, D. M., Bruce, D. R., Springer, S. A., and Friedland, G. H. (2007). Superiority of directly administered antiretroviral therapy over self-administered therapy among HIV-infected drug users: A prospective, randomized, controlled trial. *Clinical Infectious Diseases, 45,* 770–778.

American Public Health Association. (2004). *Adherence to HIV Treatment Regimens: Recommendations for Best Practices*. Washington, DC: Author.

Ammassari, A., Murri, R., Pezzotti, P., Trotta, M. P., Ravasio, L., De Longis, P., ... Antinori, A. (2001). Self-reported symptoms and medication side effects influence adherence to highly active antiretroviral therapy in persons with HIV infection. *Journal of Acquired Immune Deficiency Syndrome, 28*, 445–449.

AVERTing HIV and AIDS. (2008). *Why Is Uganda Interesting?* West Sussex, England: Author.

Badri, M., Wilson, D., & Wood, R. (2002). Effect of highly active antiretroviral therapy on incidence of tuberculosis in South Africa: A cohort study. *The Lancet, 359*, 2059–2064.

Bandura, A. (2002). Social foundations of thought and action. In D. F. Marks (Ed.), *Health Psychology Reader* (pp. 94–105). Thousand Oaks, CA: SAGE Publications.

Bangsberg, D. R., Kroetz, D. L., & Deeks, S. G. (2007). Adherence-resistance relationships to combination HIV antiretroviral therapy. *Current HIV/AIDS Reports, 4*, 65–72.

Bartlett, J. A., DeMasi, R., Quinn, J., Moxham, C., & Rousseau, F. (2001). Overview of the effectiveness of triple combination therapy in antiretroviral-naive HIV-1 infected adults. *AIDS, 15*, 1369–1377.

Bateganya, M., Colfax, C., Shafer, L. A., Kityo, C., Mugyenyi, P., Serwadda, D., ... Bangsberg, D. (2005). Antiretroviral therapy and sexual behavior: A comparative study between antiretroviral naive and experienced patients at an urban HIV/AIDS care and research center in Kampala, Uganda. *AIDS Patient Care and STDs, 19*(11), 760–768.

Becker, M. H. (1985). Patient adherence to prescribed therapies. *Medical Care, 23(5)*, 539–555.

Berg, C. J., Michelson, S. E., & Safren, S. A. (2007). Behavioral aspects of HIV care: Adherence, depression, substance use, and HIV transmission behaviors. *Infectious Disease Clinics of North America, 21*, 181–200.

Bongaarts, J. (1996). Global trends in AIDS mortality. *Population and Development Review, 22*(1), 21–45.

Bongaarts, J., Pelletier, F., & Gerland, P. (2009). Poverty, gender, and youth: Global trends in AIDS mortality. Working Paper No. 16. New York, NY: Population Council. Retrieved from http://www.popcouncil.org/pdfs/wp/pgy/016.pdf.

Boyle, B. A. (2005). Advances in HIV treatment: The 3rd International AIDS Society conference. *The AIDS Reader, 15*, 552–557.

Broder, S. (2010). The development of antiretroviral therapy and its impact on the HIV-1/AIDS pandemic. *Antiviral Research, 85*(1), 1–18.

Brownell, K., & Cohen, D. (1995). Adherence to dietary regimens. *Behavioral Medicine, 20*, 149–154.

Brunton, L. L., Lazo, J. S., and Parker, K. L. (2006) *Goodman & Gilman's The Pharmacological Basis of Therapeutics* (11th edition). New York, NY: McGraw-Hill.

Bunnell, R., Ekwaru, J. P., Solberg, P., Wamai, N., Bikaako-Kajura, W., Were, W., ... Mermin, J. (2006). Change in sexual behavior and risk of HIV transmission after antiretroviral therapy and prevention interventions in rural Uganda. *AIDS, 10*, 85–91.

Buve, A., Bishikwabo-Ssarhaza, K., & Mutangadura, G. (2002). The spread and effect of HIV-1 infection in sub-Sahara Africa. *The Lancet, 359*, 9322.

Carballo, E., Cadarso-Suárez, C., Carrera, I., Fraga, J., de la Fuente, J., Ocampo, A., ... Prieto, A. (2004). Assessing relationships between health-related quality of life and adherence to antiretroviral therapy. *Quality of Life Research, 13*, 587–599.

Cheonis, N. (2005). Immune reconstitution syndrome. *The Body*. New York, NY. Retrieved from http://www.thebody.com/content/art2525.html.

Cichocki, M. (2009). New HIV medications in 2001. About.com. Retrieved fromhttp://aids.about.com/od/studiestrials/a/newmeds_2001a.htm.

Cobb, S. (1976). Presidential address, 1976: Social support as a moderator of life stress. *Psychosomatic Medicine, 38*(5), 300–314.

Concise Medical Dictionary (7th ed.). (2008). New York, NY: Oxford University Press.

Connell, R. W. (1987). *Gender and Power*. Stanford, CA: Stanford University Press.

Cook, J. A., Grey, D., Burke, J., Cohen, M. H., Gurtman, A. C., Richardson, J. L., … Hessol, N. A. (2004). Depressive symptoms and AIDS-related among a multi-site cohort of HIV-positive women. *American Journal of Public Health, 94*, 1133–1140.

Coreil, J., Bryant, C. A., & Henderson, N. J. (2001). *Social Behavioral Foundations of Public Health*. Thousand Oaks, CA: Sage Publications.

Crepaz, N., Hart, T. A., & Marks, G. (2004). Highly active antiretroviral therapy and sexual risk behavior. *Journal of American Medical Association, 292*, 224–236.

Crosby, R. A., Kegler, M. C., & DiClemente, R. J. (2002). Understanding and applying theory in health promotion practice and research. In R. J. DiClemente, R. A. Crosby, & M. C. Kegler (Eds.), *Emerging Theories in Health Promotion Practice and Research* (pp. 1–12). San Francisco, CA: Jossey-Bass.

Daniels, N. (2005). Fair process in patient selection for antiretroviral treatment in WHO's goal of 3 by 5. *The Lancet, 366*, 9480.

de Béthune, M. (2009). Non-nucleoside reverse transcriptase inhibitors (NNRTIs), their discovery, development, and use in the treatment of

HIV-1 infection: A review of the last 20 years (1989–2009). *Antiviral Research, 85*(1), 75–90.

De Clercq, E. (2009). The history of antiretrovirals: Key discoveries over the past 25 years. *Reviews in Medical Virology, 19*(5), 287–299.

Deeks, S., Grant, R., Wrin, T., Paxinos, E., Liegler, T., Hoh, R., ... Petropoulos, C. (2003). Persistence of drug-resistant HIV-1 after a structured treatment interruption and its impact on treatment response. *AIDS, 17*(3), 361–370.

Department of Health and Human Services. (2007). HIV Treatment and the Non-Clinician: Getting Your Bearings. Rockville, MD: Author. Retrieved from http://www.ask.hrsa.gov/detail_materials.cfm?ProdID=3898.

Descamps, D. (2000). Mechanisms of Virologic Failure in Previously Untreated HIV-Infected Patients From a Trial of Induction-Maintenance Therapy. *Jama: the Journal of the American Medical Association, 283*, 2, 205–211.

DiMatteo, R. M., Lepper, H. S., & Croghan, T. W. (2000). Depression is a risk factor for non-compliance with medical treatment: Meta-analysis of the effects of anxiety and depression on patient adherence. *Archives of Internal Medicine, 160*, 2101–2107.

DiMatteo, R. M., Giordani, P. J., Lepper, H. S., & Crogham, T. W. (2002). Patient adherence and medical treatment outcomes: A meta-analysis. *Medical Care, 40*(9), 794–811.

Downes, D., & Rock, P. (2003). *Understanding Deviance: A Guide to the Sociology of Crime and Rule Breaking* (4th ed.). New York, NY: Oxford University Press.

Durkheim, E. (1951). *Suicide*. New York, NY: The Free Press. (Original work published 1897).

Essex, M., & Mboup, S. (2002). Regional variations in the African epidemics. In M. Essex, S. Mboup, P. K. Kanki, R. G. Marlink, & S. D. Tlou (Eds.), *AIDS in Africa* (2nd ed.) (pp. 90–100). New York, NY: Plenum Publishers.

Esu-Williams, E., & Blancard, K. (2002). Female condoms and microbicides. In M. Essex, S. Mboup, P. K. Kanki, R. G. Marlink, & S. D. Tlou (Eds.), *AIDS in Africa* (2nd ed.) (pp. 507–513). New York, NY: Plenum Publishers.

Fannin, S., Gottlieb, M. S., & Weisman, J. D. (1982). An outbreak of pneumocystis jiroveci pneumonia with 1 predominant genotype among renal transplant recipients: Interhuman transmission or a common environmental source? *Clinicals of Infectious Diseases, 44*(9), 1143–1149.

Farinpour, R., Miller, E. N., Satz, P., Selnes, O. A., Cohen, B. A., Becker, J. T., ... Visscher, B. R. (2003). Psychosocial risk factors of HIV morbidity and mortality: Findings from the Multi-Center AIDS Cohort Study (MACS). *Journal of Clinical and Experimental Neuropsychology, 25*, 654–670.

Ferradini, L., Jeannin, A., Pinoges, L., Izopet, J., Odhiambo, D., Mankhambo, L., ... Brasher, C. (2006). Scaling up of highly antiretroviral therapy in a rural district in Malawi. *The Lancet, 367*, 1335–1342.

Flexner, C. (2007). HIV drug development: The next 25 years. *Nature Reviews Drug Discovery, 6*, 959–966.

Food and Agriculture Organization. (2002). *Living Well With HIV: A Manual on Nutritional Care and Support for People Living With HIV*. Rome, Italy: Author.

Food and Agriculture Organization. (2008). *The Numbers: SOFI 2004 Hunger Statistics*. Budapest, Hungary: Author.

Gao, X., Nau, D. P., Rosenbluth, S. A., Scott, V., & Woodward, C. (2000). The relationship of disease severity, health beliefs and medication adherence among HIV patients. *AIDS Care, 12*(4), 387–398.

Garcia, F., de Lazzari, E., Plana, M., Castro, P., Mestre, G., Nomdedeu, M., ... Gatell, J. M. (2004). Long-term CD4+ T-cell response to highly active antiretroviral therapy according to baseline CD4+ T-cell count. *Journal of Acquired Immune Deficiency Syndromes, 36*(2), 702–713.

Garcia, P. R., & Cote, J. K. (2003). Factors affecting adherence to antiretroviral therapy in people living with HIV/AIDS. *Journal of the Association of Nurses in Aids Care, 14*(4), 37–45.

Giles, S., & Brennan, E. (2001). Home nursing of HIV-positive clients. *The Canadian Nurse, 97*(1), 33.

GlaxoSmithKline. (2008). HIV medications. GlaxoSmithKline. Retrieved from www.TreatHIV.com.

Grant, R. M., Hecht, F. M., Warmerdam, M., Liu, L., Liegler, T., Petropoulos, C. J., … Kahn, J. O. (2002). Time trends in primary HIV-1 drug resistance among recently infected persons. *Journal of American Medical Association, 288*, 181–188.

Gordillo, V., Del Amo, J., Soriano, V., and Gonzalez-Lahoz, J. (1999). Sociodemographic and psychological variables influencing adherence to antiretroviral therapy. *AIDS, 13*, 1763–1769.

Gottlieb, M. S. (1981). *Pneumocystis* pneumonia—Los Angeles. *Morbidity and Mortality Weekly Report 30*(21), 1–3.

Gouws, E. (2008). The epidemiology of HIV infection among young people aged 15–24 years in southern Africa. *AIDS, 22*(4), 5–16.

Haisch, J., & Hornung, R. (2005). Perceptions, cognitions, and decisions. In J. Kerr, R. Weitkunat, & M. Moretti (Eds.), *ABC of Behavioral Change: A Guide to Successful Disease Prevention and Health Promotion* (pp. 85–97). New York, NY: Elsavier.

Halkitis, P., Palamar, J., & Mukherjee, P. (2008). Analysis of HIV medication adherence in relation to person and treatment characteristics using hierarchical linear modeling. *AIDS Patient Care and STDs, 22*(4), 323–335.

Hammer, S. M., Saag, M. S., Schechter, M., Montaner, J. S. G., Schooley, R. T., Jacobsen, D. M., … Volberding, P. A. (2006). Treatment for adult HIV infection: 2006 recommendations of the International AIDS

Society–USA panel. *Journal of American Medical Association, 296*, 827–843.

Hanson, K., & Hicks, C. (2006). New antiretroviral drugs. *Current HIV/AIDS Reports, 3*(2), 93–101.

Hardeman, W., Johnston, M., Johnston, D. W., Bonetti, D., Wareman, N. J., & Kinmonth, A. L. (2002). Application of the theory of planned behaviors in behavior change interventions: A systematic review. *Psychology and Health, 17*, 123–158.

Harden, V. A. (1992). Koch's postulates and the etiology of AIDS: An historical perspective. *History and Philosophy of the Life Sciences, 14*(2), 249–269.

Hardon, A. P., Akurut, D., Comoro, C., Ekezie, C., Irunde, H. F., Gerrits, T., … Laing, R. (2007). Hunger, waiting time and transport costs: Time to confront challenges to ART adherence in Africa. *AIDS Care, 19*(5), 658–665.

Hardon, A. P., Aurugai, D. A., Comoro, C., Ekezie, C., Irunde, H., Gerrits, T., … Laing, R. (2006). On hunger, transport costs and waiting time: A synthesis of challenges to ARV drugs adherence in three African countries. In S. Davy (Ed.), *Access to Adherence, the Challenges of Antiretroviral Treatment* (pp. 15–36). Geneva, Switzerland: World Health Organization. Retrieved from http://apps.who.int/medicinedocs/pdf/s13400e/s13400e.pdf.

Harrigan, P. R., Hogg, R. S., Dong, W. W. Y., Yip, B., Wynhoven, B., Woodward, J., … Montaner, J. S. G. (2005). Predictors of HIV drug-resistance mutations in a large antiretroviral-naive cohort initiating triple antiretroviral therapy. *Journal of Infectious Diseases, 191*(3), 339–347.

Haubrich, R. H., Little, S. J., Currier, J. S., Forthal, D. N., Kemper, C. A., Beall, G. N., … McCutchan, J. A. (1999). The value of patient-reported adherence to antiretroviral therapy in predicting virologic and immunologic response. *AIDS, 13*, 1099–1107.

HIV Clinical Resource. (2007). Antiretroviral therapy. New York State Department of Health AIDS Institute. Retrieved from http://www.hivguidelines.org.

Hogg, R. S., Heath, K., Bangsberg, D., Yip, B., Press, N., O'Shaughnessy, M. V., & Montaner, J. S. G. (2002). Intermittent use of triple-combination therapy is predictive of mortality at baseline and after 1 year of follow-up. *AIDS, 16*, 1051–1058.

Holwerda, V. L. (2000). The health belief model and self breast examination in nurses. (Unpublished doctoral dissertation). Grand Valley State University, Allendale, MI.

Holzemer, W. L., Corless, I. B., Nokes, K. M., Turner, J. G., Brown, M. A., Powell-Cope, G. M., … Portillo, C. J. (1999). Predictors of self-reported adherence in persons living with HIV disease. *AIDS Patient Care STDS, 13*(3), 185–197.

Jelsma, J., Maclean, E., Hughes, J., Tinese, X., & Darder, M. (2005). An investigation into the health-related quality of life of individuals living with HIV who are receiving HAART. *AIDS Care, 17*(5), 579–588.

Kalichman, S. C., Ramachandran, B., & Catz, S. (1999). Adherence to combination antiretroviral therapies in HIV patients of low health literacy. *Journal of General Internal Medicine, 14*, 267–273.

Kalichman, S. C., Rompa, D., DiFonzo, K., Simpson, D., Austin, J., Luke, W., … Buckles, J. (2001). HIV treatment adherence in women living with HIV/AIDS: Research based on the information-motivation-behavioral skills model of health behavior. *The Journal of the Association of Nurses in AIDS Care, 12*(4), 58–67.

Keller, C., Fleury, J., Gregor-Holt, N., & Thompson, T. (1999). Predictive ability of social cognitive theory in exercise research: An integrated literature review. *Online Journal of Knowledge Synthesis for Nursing, 6*(2). Retrieved from http://www.des.emory.edu/mfp/KellerEtAl1999.pdf.

Kerbo, H. R. (2003). *Social Stratification and Inequality: Class Conflict in Historical, Comparative, and Global Perspective* (5th ed.). New York, NY: McGraw Hill.

Kerr, J., Weitkunat, R., & Moretti, M. (Eds.). (2005). *ABC of Behavioral Change: A Guide to Successful Disease Prevention and Health Promotion.* New York, NY: Elsavier.

Kitahata, M. M., Reed, S. D., Dillingham, P. W., Van Rompaey, S. E., Young, A. A., Harrington, D. R., & Holmes, K. K. (2004). Pharmacy-based assessment of adherence to HAART predicts virologic and immunologic treatment response and clinical progression to AIDS and death. *International Journal of STD & AIDS, 15*(12), 803–810.

Komiti, A., Judd, F., Grech, P., Mijch, A., Hoy, J., Williams, B., ... Lloyd, J. H. (2003). Depression in people living with HIV/AIDS attending primary care and outpatient clinics. *Australian and New Zealand Journal of Psychiatry, 37*, 70–77.

Krishnan, A. K. S., Hendricksen, E., Vallabhaneni, S., Johnson, S. L., Raminani, S. N., Kumarasamy, N., ... Safren, S. A. (2007). Sexual behaviors of individuals with HIV living in south India: A qualitative study. *AIDS Education and Prevention, 19*(4), 334–345.

Laing, R., & Hodgkin, C. (2006). Overview of antiretroviral therapy, adherence and drug resistance. In A. Hardon et al. (Eds.), *From Access to Adherence, the Challenges of Antiretroviral Treatment: Studies From Botswana, Tanzania and Uganda* (pp. 21–31). Geneva, Switzerland: World Health Organization.

Last, J. M. (Ed.). (2007). *Dictionary of Public Health* (1st ed.). New York, NY: Oxford University Press.

Leventhal, H., & Cameron, L. (1987). Behavioral theories and the problem of compliance. *Patient Education and Counseling, 10*(2), 117–138.

Liska, A. E., & Messner, S. F. (1999). *Perspectives on Crime and Deviance* (3rd ed.). Upper Saddle River, NJ: Prentice Hall.

Lohse, N., Hansen, A.-B. E., Gerstoft, J., & Obel, N. (2007). Improved survival in HIV-infected persons: consequences and perspectives. *Journal of Antimicrobial Chemotherapy, 60*, 461–463.

Lucas, G. M., Chaisson, R. E., & Moore, R. D. (1999). Highly active antiretroviral therapy in a large urban clinic: Risk factors for virologic failure and adverse drug reactions. *Annals of Internal Medicine, 131*(2), 81–87.

Lucas, G. M. (2005). Antiretroviral adherence, drug resistance, viral fitness and HIV disease progression: A tangled web is woven. *Journal of Antimicrobial Chemotherapy, 55*, 413–416.

Luszczynska, A., & Sutton, S. (2005). Attitudes and expectations. In J. Kerr, R. Weitkunat, & M. Moretti (Eds.), *ABC of Behavioral Change: A Guide to Successful Disease Prevention and Health Promotion* (pp. 71–84). New York, NY: Elsavier.

Machtinger, E. L., & Bangsberg, D. R. (2008). *Adherence to HIV Antiretroviral Therapy*. San Francisco, CA: University of California: HIV InSite, UCSF Center for HIV Information.

Mannheimer, S., Friedland, G., Matts, J., Child, C., & Chesney, M. (2002). The consistency of adherence to antiretroviral therapy predicts biologic outcomes for human immunodeficiency virus-infected persons in clinical trials. *Clinical Infectious Diseases, 34*(8), 1115–1121.

Mannheimer, S. B., Matts, J., Telzak, E., Chesney, M., Child, C., Wu, A. W., & Friedland, G. (2005). Quality of life in HIV-infected individuals receiving antiretroviral therapy is related to adherence. *AIDS Care, 17*(1), 10–22.

McNicholl, I. (2007). *Adverse Effects of Antiretroviral Drugs*. San Francisco, CA: HIV InSite, UCSF Center for HIV Information.

Melbourne, K. M., Geletko, S. M., Brown, S. L., Willey-Lessne, C., Chase, S., & Fisher, A. (1999). Medication adherence in patients with HIV infection: A comparison of two measurement methods. *AIDS Reader, 9*(5), 329–338.

Mills, E. J., Nachega, J. B., Buchan, I., Orbinski, J., Attaran, A., Singh, S., … Bangsberg, D. R. (2006). Adherence to antiretroviral therapy in sub-Saharan Africa and North America. *The Journal of the American Medical Association, 296*(6), 679–690.

Mirowsky, J., Ross, C. E., & Reynolds, J. (2000). Links between social status and health. In C. E. Bird, P. Conrad, & A. M. Fremont (Eds.), *The Handbook of Medical Sociology* (5th ed.) (pp. 47–67). Upper Saddle River, NJ: Prentice Hall.

Moatti, J. P., Carrieri, M. P., Spire, B., Gastaut, J. A., Cassuto, J. P., & Moreau, J. (2000). Adherence to HAART in French HIV infected injecting drug users: The contribution of buprenorphine drug maintenance treatment. *AIDS, 14*, 151–155.

Mocroft, A., Phillips, A. N., Gatell, J., Ledergerber, B., Fisher, M., Clumeck, N., … Lundgren, J. D. (2007). Normalization of CD4 counts in patients with HIV-1 infection and maximum virological suppression who are taking combination antiretroviral therapy: An observational cohort study. *The Lancet, 370*(9585), 407–413.

Morbidity and Mortality Weekly Report. (2003). Advancing HIV prevention: New strategies for a changing epidemic. *Morbidity and Mortality Report, 52*(15), 329–434.

Moyer, T. P., Temesgen, Z., Enger, R., Estes, L., Charlson, J., Oliver, L., & Wright, A. (1999). Drug monitoring of antiretroviral therapy for HIV-1 infection: Method validation and resultants of a pilot study. *Clinical Chemistry, 45*, 1465–1476.

MSUCARES. (2001). Health education behavior models and theories—A review of the literature—Part I. Mississippi State University Extension Service Coordinated Access to Research and Extension System (MSU-CARES). Retrieved from http://msucares.com/health/health/appa1.htm.

Mugyenyi, P., Kityo, C., Kibende, S., Ssali, F., Kabuye, G., Otim, T., … Kabugo, M. (2006). Scaling up antiretroviral therapy: Experience of the Joint Clinical Research Center (JCRC) access program. *Acta Academica Supplementum, 1*, 216–240.

Munro, S., Lewin, S., Swart, T., & Volmink, J. (2007). A review of health behavior theories: How useful are these for developing interventions to promote long-term medication adherence for TB and HIV/AIDS. BioMed Central. Retrieved from http://www.biomedcentral.com/1471-2458/7/104.

Northwestern Memorial Hospital. (2008). HIV/AIDS. Chicago, IL: Northwestern Memorial Hospital. Retrieved from http://www.nmh.org/nm/infectious-disease-hiv.

Palella, F. J., Delaney, K. M., Moorman, A. C., Loveless, M. O., Fuhrer, J., Satten, G. A., … Holmberg, S. D. (1998). Declining morbidity and mortality among patients with advanced human immunodeficiency virus infection. *The New England Journal of Medicine, 338*(13), 853–860.

Panel on Antiretroviral Guidelines for Adult and Adolescents. (2011). Guidelines for the use of antiretroviral agents in HIV-1-infected adults and adolescents. Department of Health and Human Services. Retrieved from http://www.aidsinfo.nih.gov/contentfiles/adultandadolescentgl.pdf.

Park, D. C., & Mayhorn, C. B. (1996). Remembering to take medications: The importance of non-memory variables. In D. Herrmann, C. Envoy, C. Hertzog, P. Hertel, & M. K. Johnson (Eds.), *Basic and Applied Memory Research: Practical Applications Volume 2* (pp. 90–101). Hillsdale, NJ: Lawrence Erlbaum.

Parsons, T. (1951). *The Social System.* London: Routledge and Kegan Press.

Paterson, D. L., Swindells, S., Mohr, J., Brester, M., Vergis, E. N., Squier, C., … Singh, N. (2000). Adherence of protease inhibitor therapy and outcomes in patients with HIV infection. *Annals of Internal Medicine, 133*(1), 21–30.

Petosa, R., & Jackson, K. (1991). Using the health belief model to predict safer sex intentions among adolescents. *Health Education & Behavior, 18*(4), 463–476.

Prentice-Dunn, S., & Rogers, R. W. (1986). Protection motivation theory and preventive health: Beyond the health belief model. *Health Education Research, 1*(3), 153–161.

Pulerwitz, J., Amaro, H., De Jong, W., Gortmaker, S. L., & Rudd, R. (2002). Relationship power, condom use and HIV risk among women in the USA. *AIDS Care, 14*(6), 789–800.

Redding, C. A., Rossi, J. S., Rossi, S. R., Velicer, W. F., & Prochaska, J. O. (2000). Health behavior models. *The International Electronic Journal of Health Education—Special Issue 3*, 180–193. Retrieved from http://drzaius.ics.uci.edu/meta/classes/informatics161_fall06/papers/10a-Redding_HealthBehaviorModels.pdf.

Remien, R. H., Exner, T. M., Morin, S. F., Ehrhardt, A. A., Johnson, M. O., Correale, J., ... the NIMH Healthy Living Project Team. (2007). Medication adherence and sexual risk behavior among HIV-infected adults: Implications for transmission of resistant virus. *Journal of AIDS and Behavior, 11*(5), 663–675.

Rieker, P. P., & Bird, C. E. (2000). Sociological explanations of gender differences in mental and physical health. In C. E. Bird, P. Conrad, & A. M. Fremont, *Handbook of Medical Sociology* (5th ed.) (pp. 98–113). Upper Saddle River, NJ: Prentice Hall.

Robbins, R. H. (2005). *Global Problems and the Culture of Capitalism.* New York, NY: Pearson Education, Inc.

Rogers, R. W. (1975). A protection motivation theory of fear appeals and attitude change. *Journal of Psychology, 91*, 93–114.

Rosenstock, I. M. (1974). The health belief model and preventative health behavior. *Health Education Monographs, 2*, 354–386.

Rowell, P., & Shippy, R. (2004). What a difference a decade made: Quality of life in adults living with HIV/AIDS. *The Gerontologist, 648.*

Sa, Z., & Larsen, U. (2006). Gender inequality and HIV-1 infection among women in Moshi, Tanzania. Paper presented at the annual meeting of the American Sociological Association, Montreal Convention Center, Montreal, Quebec, Canada.

San Francisco AIDS Foundation. (2007). Treatment. Retrieved from http://www.sfaf.org/aids101/treatment.html#antiviral.

Safren, S. A., Kumarasamy, N., James, R., Raminani, S., Solomon, S., & Mayer, K. H. (2005). ART adherence, demographic variables and CD4 outcome among HIV positive patients on antiretroviral therapy in Chennai, India. *AIDS Care, 17*(7), 853–862.

Samet, J. H., Libman, H., Steger, K. A., Dhawan, R. K., Chen, J., Shevitz, A. H., … Craven, D. E. (1992). Compliance with zidovudine therapy in patients infected with human immunodeficiency virus, type 1: A cross-sectional study in a municipal hospital clinic. *The American Journal of Medicine, 92*(5), 495–502.

Saunders, J. (2000). *Top Drugs: Top Synthetic Routes*. New York, NY: Oxford University Press.

Schmitt, S. K., & Mehta, N. (2002). Systematic reviews of infectious diseases. *Clinical Infectious Diseases, 34*, 1515–1523.

Sen, S., Mathur, A. G., Gupta, R. M., Kapila, K., & Chopra, G. S. (2008). Investigational antiretroviral drugs. *Recent Patents on Anti-Infective Drug Discovery, 3*(3), 199–205.

Schonneson, L. L., Williams, M. L., Ross, M. W., Diamond, P. M., & Keel, B. (2007). Three types of adherence to HIV antiretroviral therapy and their association with AIDS diagnosis, medication, side effects, beliefs about antiretroviral therapy, and beliefs about HIV disease. *International Journal of Sexually Transmitted Diseases and AIDS, 18*, 369–373.

Schwartlander, B., Grubb, I., & Perriens, J. (2006). The 10-year struggle to provide antiretroviral treatment to people with HIV in the developing world. *The Lancet, 368*, 541–546.

Schwartlander, B., Stover, J., Walker, N., Bollinger, L., Guterez, P., McGreevey, W., … Bertozzi, S. (2001). Resource needs for HIV/AIDS. *Science New Series, 292*(5526), 2434–2436.

Siliciano, R. (2000). Can antiretroviral therapy ever be stopped? *AIDS Reader, 10*(4), 224–229.

Singh, N., Berman, S. M., Swindells, S., Justis, J. C., Mohr, J. A., Squier, C., & Wagener, M. M. (1999). Adherence of human immunodeficiency virus-infected patients to antiretroviral therapy. *Clinical Infectious Diseases, 29*, 824–830.

Singh, N., Squier, C., Sivek, C., Wagener, M., Nguyen, M. H., & Yu, V. L. (1996). Determinants of compliance antiretroviral therapy in patients with human immunodeficiency virus: Prospective assessment with implications for enhancing compliance. *AIDS Care, 8*, 261–269.

Sterling, T. R., Chaisson, R. E., Keruly, J., & Moore, R. D. (2003). Improved outcomes with earlier initiation of highly active antiretroviral therapy among human immunodeficiency virus–infected patients who achieve durable virologic suppression: Longer follow-up of an observational cohort study. *The Journal of Infectious Diseases, 188*, 1659–1665.

Tarby, C. M. (2004). Recent advances in the development of next generation non-nucleoside reverse transcriptase inhibitors. *Current Topics in Medicinal Chemistry, 4*(10), 1045–1057.

Uganda Ministry of Health & ORC Marco. (2006). Uganda HIV/AIDS sero-behavioral survey 2004–2005. Calverton, MD: Author.

UNAIDS. (2006a). *Treatment and Care*. Geneva, Switzerland: Author.

UNAIDS. (2006b). *2006 Report on the Global AIDS Epidemic: A UNAIDS 10th Anniversary Special Edition*. Geneva, Switzerland: Author.

UNAIDS. (2006c). *2006 Report on the Global AIDS Epidemic*. Geneva, Switzerland: Author.

UNAIDS. (2009). *Annual Report 2009*. Geneva, Switzerland: Author.

UNAIDS. (2010a). *UNAIDS Report on the Global AIDS Epidemic 2010*. Geneva, Switzerland: Author.

UNAIDS. (2010b). *Financing the Response to AIDS in Low- and Middle-Income Countries: International Assistance from the G8, European Commission and Other Donor Governments in 2009*. Geneva, Switzerland: Author.

U.S. Department of State. (2004). *The President's Emergency Plan for AIDS Relief: U.S. Five-Year Global HIV/AIDS Strategy*. Washington, DC: Author.

U.S. Department of State. (2007). *Uganda FY 2007 Country Operational Plan (COP)*. Washington, DC: Author.

U.S. Department of State. (2008). *Bureau of African Affairs January 2008*. Washington, DC: Author. Retrieved from http://www.state.gov/r/pa/ei/bgn/2963.htm.

U.S. Department of State. (2011). *PEPFAR Funding: Investments That Save Lives and Promote Security*. Washington, DC: Author.

U.S. Global AIDS Coordinator. (2008). *The Power of Partnerships: Fourth Annual Report to Congress on PEPFAR*. Washington, DC. Retrieved from http://www.pepfar.gov/press/fourth_annual_report/.

Vanhove, G., Schapiro, J., Winters, M. A., Merigan, T. C., & Blaschke, T. F. (1996). Patient adherence and drug failure in protease inhibitor monotherapy. *Journal of American Medical Association, 276*, 1955–1956.

Weber, M. (2002). *The Protestant Ethic and the Spirit of Capitalism*. (S. Kalberg, Trans.). Los Angeles, CA: Roxbury Publishing Company.

WebMD. (2008). Human immunodeficiency virus. New York, NY: MedicineNet. Retrieved from http://www.medicinenet.com/human_immunodeficiency_virus_hiv_aids/article.htm.

Weidle, P. J., Wamai, N., Solberg, P., Liechty, C., Sendagala, S., Were, W., … Bunnell, R. (2006). Adherence to antiretroviral therapy in a home-based AIDS care programme in rural Uganda. *Lancet, 368*(9547):1587–1594.

Weidle, P. J., Malamb, S., Mwebaze, R., & Sozi, C. (2002). Assessment of a pilot antiretroviral drug therapy programme in Uganda, patients' response, survival, and drug resistance. *The Lancet, 360*, 9326.

Weinberg, M. A., & Friedland, G. (1998). Public health implications of antiretroviral therapy and HIV drug resistance. *Journal of the American Medical Association, 279*, 1977–1983.

Weiss, G. L., & Lonnquist, L. E. (2003). *The Sociology of Health, Healing, and Illness* (4th ed.). Upper Saddle River, NJ: Prentice Hall.

Wensing, A., & Boucher, C. (2003). Worldwide transmission of drug-resistant HIV. *AIDS, 5*, 140–155.

Williams, A., & Friedland, G. (1997). Adherence, compliance, and HAART. *AIDS Clinical Care, 9*(7), 51–54.

Wilson, T. E., Barron, Y., Cohen, M., Richardson, J., Greenblatt, R., Sacks, H. S., & Young, M. (2002). Adherence to antiretroviral therapy and its association with sexual behavior in a national sample of women with human immunodeficiency virus. *Clinical Infectious Diseases, 34*, 529–534.

Wingood, G. M., & DiClemente, R. J. (2000). Application of the theory of gender and power to examine HIV-related exposures, risk factors, and effective interventions for women. *Health Education and Behavior, 27*(5), 539–565. Retrieved from http://heb.sagepub.com/cgi/content/abstract/27/5/539.

Wood, E., Hogg, R., Yip, B., Harrigan, R., O'Shaughnessey, M. V., & Montaner, J. S. G. (2003). Effect of medication adherence on survival of HIV-infected adults who start highly active antiretroviral therapy when the CD4+ cell count is 200 to 350. *Annals of Internal Medicine, 139*(10), 810–816.

World Bank. (2011). *Data: Poverty*. Washington, DC: Author.

World Health Organization. (2003a). *Scaling Up Antiretroviral Therapy in Resource-Limited Settings: Treatment Guidelines for a Public Health*

Approach. Geneva, Switzerland: Author. Retrieved from http://www.who.int/3by5/publications/documents/arv_guidelines/en/index.html.

World Health Organization. (2003b). *Adherence to Long Term Therapies: Evidence for Action*. Geneva, Switzerland: Author.

World Health Organization. (2004). *Treat 3 Million by 2005: Scaling Up Antiretroviral Therapy in Resource-Limited Settings—Treatment Guidelines for a Public Health Approach*. Geneva, Switzerland: Author.

World Health Organization. (2006a). *Progress In Scaling Up Access to HIV Treatment in Low and Middle Income Countries*. Geneva, Switzerland: Author.

World Health Organization. (2006b). *Towards Universal Access by 2010*. Geneva, Switzerland: Author.

World Health Organization. (2006c). *Progress on Global Access to HIV Antiretroviral Therapy: A Report On 3 X 5 and Beyond March 2006*. Geneva, Switzerland: Author. Retrieved from http://www.who.int/hiv/progressreport2006_en.pdf.

World Health Organization. (2008a). *HIV/AIDS Epidemiological Surveillance Report for the WHO African Region 2007 Update*. Geneva, Switzerland: Author.

World Health Organization. (2008b). *Antiretroviral Treatment Failure Due To Lack Of Patient Support*. Geneva, Switzerland: Author.

World Health Organization. (2008c). *Agents in HIV-1-Infected Adults and Adolescents*. Geneva, Switzerland: Author.

World Health Organization. (2009a). *HIV Surveillance, Estimates, Monitoring and Evaluation*. Geneva, Switzerland: Author.

World Health Organization. (2011a). *Gender, Women and Health: Gender Inequalities and HIV*. Geneva, Switzerland: Author. Retrieved from http://www.who.int/3by5/publications/documents/arv_guidelines/en/index.html.

World Health Organization. (2011b). *Global Health Observatory: HIV/ AIDS*. Geneva, Switzerland: Author.

Wurth, S., & Perlow, M. (2005). Perceived barriers to adherence as described by individuals with HIV disease. *Kentucky Nurse, 53*, 1.

Yeni, P. G., Hammer, S. M., Hirsch, M. S., Saag, M. S., Schechter, M., Carpenter, C. C. J., … Volberding, P. A. (2005). Treatment for adult HIV infection: 2004 recommendations of the International AIDS Society-USA Panel. *Journal of the American Medical Association, 292*, 251–265.

Index